Gastric Sleeve Bariatric Cookbook

The Comprehensive Guide to Easy & Delicious

Post-Surgery Meal Plans & Recipes

(Quick Prep Tips Included)

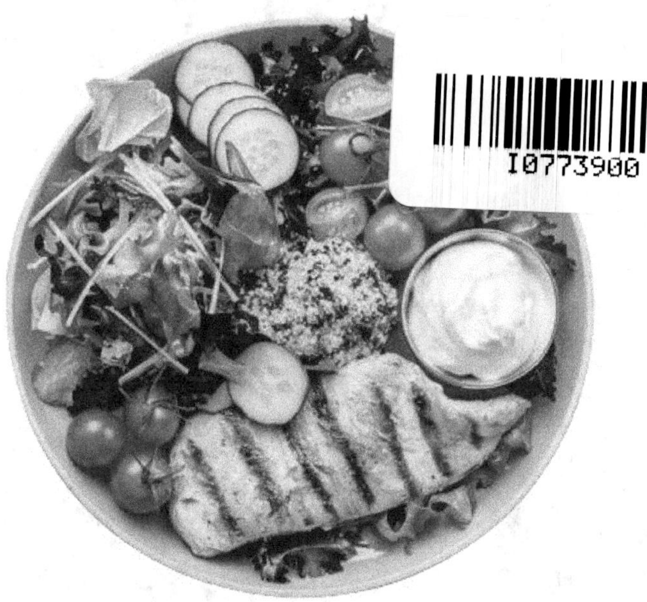

Catherine D Crisp

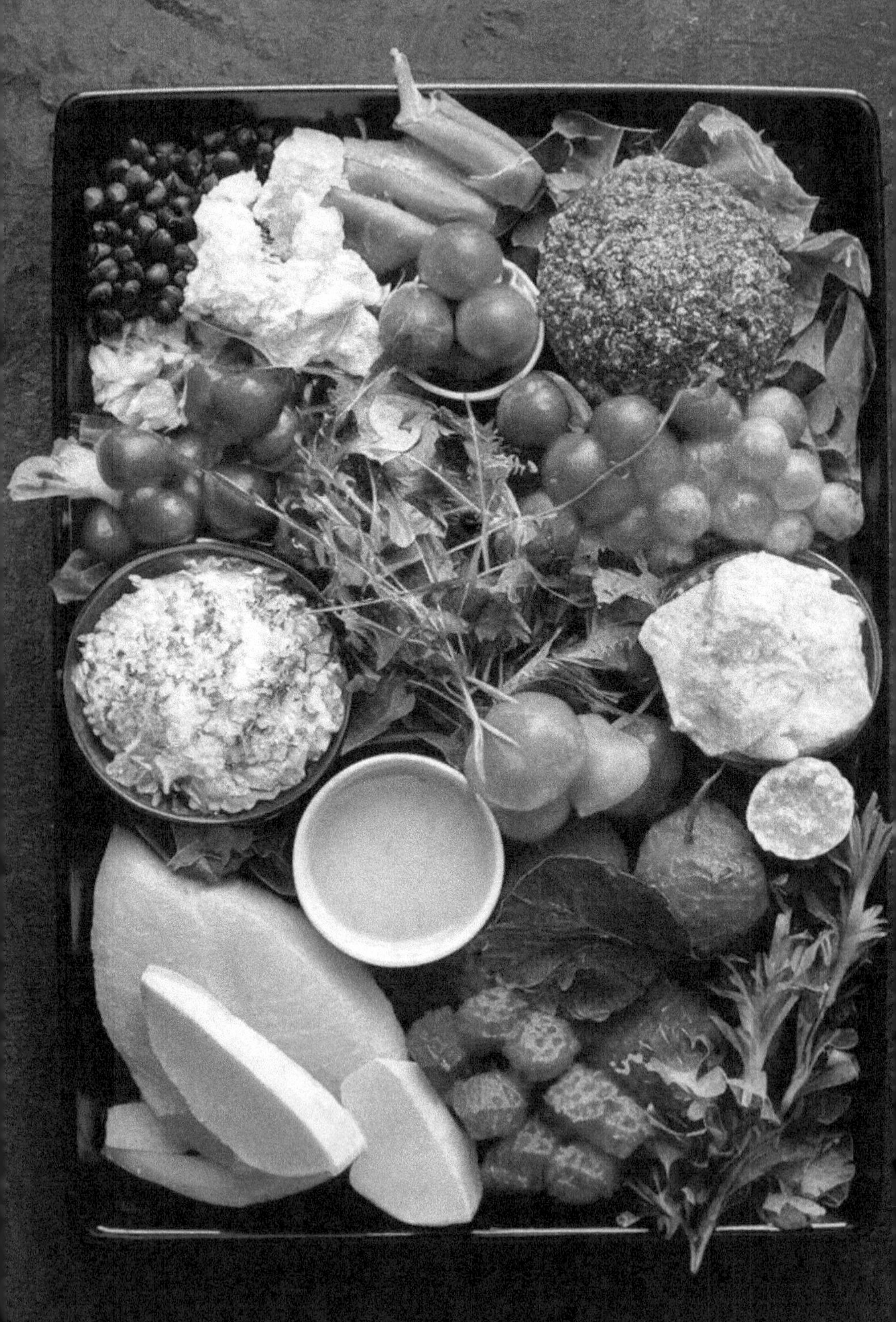

Disclaimer

The information in the book is based on personal research and experience. The author advises readers to consult with their healthcare provider before making any dietary changes

For more information or to contact the author, please email: catherinecrispnutrition@gmail.com

HOW TO USE THIS BOOK

Welcome to a pivotal moment in your journey toward enhanced well-being! This book is your ally as you navigate the complexities following bariatric surgery, recognizing the blend of hope and uncertainty that characterizes this path.

Here's a structured plan to maximize the benefits from this book:

Step 1: Evaluate Your Needs and Objectives:

- **Self-reflection:** Spend some time reflecting on recent dietary, exercise, or body image challenges. Identify areas you're eager to improve.

- **Identify Priorities:** Your journey is unique. While this book provides a broad spectrum of strategies, pinpoint the essentials relevant to your current needs. Are there specific dietary plans or exercise routines you're looking for?

Step 2: Explore the Book:

- **Blueprint for Success:** Early chapters provide insights into bariatric surgery and post-operative nutrition, followed by discussions on physical activity, mental well-being, and social aspects of weight loss.

- **Seek Answers:** We've included FAQs to address common queries and obstacles encountered post-surgery.

Step 3: Tailor Your Path:

- **Customization is Key:** Feel free to mark important sections or jot notes in the margins. This guide is designed for customization to suit your journey.

- **Adjust as Needed:** The book lays down the basics of nutrition and meal planning. Adapt these to fit your taste and nutritional needs, always consulting healthcare professionals for personalized advice.

- **Diverse Learning Approaches:** Whether through text, charts, or meal plans, find the learning method that resonates with you.

Step 4: Forge Your Support Network:

- **Community Strength:** You're not alone. Beyond this guide, seek support from family, friends, and healthcare providers. Share your aspirations and challenges to bolster your support network.

- **Online Engagement:** Participate in online forums for individuals post-bariatric surgery. Sharing and receiving support can greatly enhance motivation and accountability.

Step 5: Embrace the Journey:

- **Celebrate Progress:** Focus on ongoing improvement rather than perfection. Embrace the small victories and maintain consistent progress.

- **Attune to Your Body:** Pay attention to hunger cues and the impacts of various foods. Adjust your eating habits to align with your body's signals.

- **Honor Your Experience:** This journey is as much emotional as it is physical. Welcome the changes and celebrate the process of rediscovering yourself.

Consider this book your guide, but remember, the real adventure lies ahead. Armed with the right tools, knowledge, and a supportive community, you can achieve lasting success and embrace a joyful, healthier life.

Let's embark on this journey together!

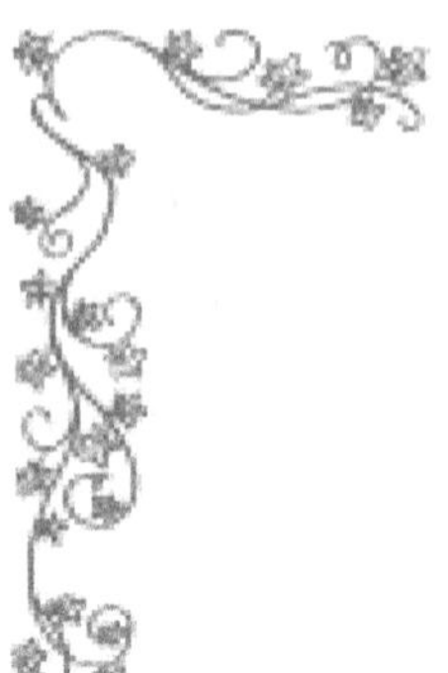

Appreciation

Hey there,

I'm really moved that you chose my book from so many options out there. It means the absolute world to me. I hope as you turn these pages, you find not just advice and guidance but also a companion. Embarking on this path shows incredible courage, and I want you to know I'm right here with you, rooting for you at every step. Here's to the journey ahead, with all its highs and lows, triumphs and lessons. I'm honored to be a part of your remarkable journey towards a healthier and happier life.

Warmest wishes,

Catherine D. Crisp

Table of Contents

CHAPTER 5

PHASE 4: THE SOFT FOODS DIET **123**

BONUS CHAPTER

10 EASY HERBAL TINCTURES & SMOOTHIES TO SPEED UP YOUR RECOVERY..................... **157**

Introduction

Over recent years, the landscape of weight loss surgery has dramatically shifted, with the sleeve gastrectomy quickly rising to prominence. This method, often referred to simply as "the sleeve," has eclipsed traditional surgeries like the Roux-en-Y gastric bypass and the adjustable gastric band, capturing the interest of individuals seeking a definitive solution to long-standing weight struggles. Sleeve gastrectomy is more than a procedure; it's a vital tool that empowers people burdened by obesity or related health issues to reclaim their lives, offering a chance for significant and swift weight reduction.

Achieving lasting success post-operation demands a deep commitment to a diet that's carefully tailored to the unique needs of a changed digestive system. It's a journey towards wellness that goes far beyond mere weight loss, aiming for a holistic improvement in health.

The digital age brings with it an abundance of information, with a simple online search about post-surgery diets yielding an overwhelming array of advice. Recognizing the need for clear, direct guidance, I was inspired to craft a cookbook that cuts through the clutter, providing essential eating guidelines for the post-operative phase. This new edition builds on that foundation, specifically catering to those who have undergone or are considering the sleeve, featuring meal plans for the crucial early weeks of recovery.

This book isn't just a collection of recipes; it's a companion on your journey to a new you. It addresses the emotional and physical aspects of post-surgery life, aiming to be a source of comfort and inspiration.

Celebrating your courageous decision to pursue a healthier lifestyle, this book acknowledges the significant step you've taken towards a lasting transformation. By opting for surgery, you've employed the most effective strategy available for achieving your health goals. This decision marks the end of frustrating diet cycles and heralds a future filled with vitality and wellness. Together, let's navigate this journey, starting with practical dietary principles and exploring a world of flavorful, nourishing meals.

Welcome to your new beginning.

Chapter 1

What Is the Vertical Sleeve Gastrectomy?

Are you tired of the endless battle with weight loss and its toll on your health? Many have found a beacon of hope in Vertical Sleeve Gastrectomy (VSG), a procedure that's winning hearts for its effectiveness and simplicity compared to other weight-loss surgeries.

Picture this: a life where hunger doesn't dictate your day, and a smaller stomach naturally limits your portions. That's the reality VSG offers. It's like hitting the reset button on your stomach, removing around 75-80% of it and leaving behind a slender sleeve that curbs your appetite and kickstarts your weight loss journey. Plus, it tweaks the hormones that signal hunger and satisfaction, helping you feel full faster and cut down on your overall food intake.

So, what sets VSG apart from the rest? It's all about what doesn't happen – there's no rerouting of your intestines. Your body continues to absorb nutrients just as it always has, which means you're less likely to face nutritional deficiencies post-surgery. Of course, embracing a nutritious diet and supplementing wisely remains key to recovery.

One of the standout perks of VSG is the drop in hunger pangs. By removing the stomach's section that pumps out the hunger hormone ghrelin, your desire to snack diminishes. Combine that with your newly downsized stomach, and you've got a recipe for substantial, enduring weight loss.

Another plus? VSG is less complex than many other bariatric options. This generally translates to a smoother surgery and a quicker path to getting back on your feet.

But let's be clear: VSG isn't a one-stop solution. It's a mighty ally, but the real victory in weight loss comes from your dedication to a new, healthier way of life. Sticking to the diet plan your doctor lays out, staying active, and keeping up with your medical check-ins are the pillars of success. This holistic strategy is what makes the surgery work its magic, ensuring you shed those pounds and elevate your health for the long haul.

If obesity and its associated health woes have been weighing you down, VSG might just be the game-changer you need. It's not just about shrinking your stomach; it's about reshaping your relationship with food and hunger.

Advantages of Gastric Sleeve Surgery

- **A Tailored Approach to Portion Control:** VSG offers a physical modification that serves as a built-in portion control, reducing the stomach's volume by approximately 75-80%. This newly shaped 'sleeve' isn't just smaller; it's a constant, gentle reminder that less is more when it comes to meal sizes.

- **Harmony with Hormones:** The surgery strategically removes the part of the stomach that secretes ghrelin, the so-called 'hunger hormone.' This leads to a natural suppression of appetite, making it easier for patients to adhere to healthier eating habits without the constant battle against cravings.

- **Nutrient Absorption Remains Intact:** By avoiding any alteration to the intestinal tract, VSG maintains the body's ability to absorb nutrients effectively. This crucial aspect means that, post-surgery, patients can continue to benefit from the vitamins and minerals in their food, provided they maintain a balanced diet.

- **A Significant Stride in Weight Loss:** VSG is not just about immediate results; it's a catalyst for long-term weight management. The surgery sets the stage for a sustainable weight loss journey, helping patients achieve and maintain their goals through a combination of reduced intake and hormonal balance.

- **Health Rejuvenation:** The ripple effect of weight loss from VSG extends to a broad spectrum of health improvements. Conditions often associated with obesity, such as type 2 diabetes, hypertension, and obstructive sleep apnea, can see remarkable progress, sometimes even leading to complete remission.

- **Surgical Simplicity:** Compared to other bariatric surgeries, VSG is less invasive. This simplicity translates to a lower risk profile, potentially fewer complications, and a quicker return to daily activities, making it a compelling option for those seeking a safer surgical route.

- **Life beyond the Scale:** The benefits of VSG go beyond the numbers on the scale. Patients often report enhanced mobility, a boost in self-confidence, and a newfound zest for life. Social interactions become more enjoyable, and many embrace activities they previously avoided or found challenging.

- **A Commitment to Change:** VSG is a powerful tool, but it's the patient's commitment to a new lifestyle that truly seals the deal. A balanced diet, regular exercise, and consistent follow-up care form the triumvirate of success, ensuring the effects of the surgery are not just temporary but a gateway to a healthier future.

Tips for Recovering quickly from the Surgery

Embarking on the journey of gastric sleeve surgery is like setting sail on a new chapter of your life. It's a time filled with change, and how you navigate the post-op waters can really shape your recovery and the quality of your new life. Here's a little guide to help you steer towards smoother seas:

- **Stock Up on Essentials:** Before you even head to the hospital, make sure you've got a stash of medical must-haves. Bandages, cotton balls, pain relief meds, and heating pads should be at the ready to make your post-surgery days as comfortable as possible.

- **Wardrobe Wonders:** As you shed those extra pounds, clothes that once felt snug may suddenly feel like cozy pajamas. Before you hit the stores, it's time for a fun wardrobe excavation! Dig through drawers and forgotten corners – you might unearth hidden gems you haven't worn in ages.

- **Mindful Munching:** Overeating post-op is a no-go—it'll lead to discomfort and the dreaded return of your last meal. Slow down at the dinner table, chew thoroughly, and start with smaller portions. Skip the straws and dry snacks, and take your time with each bite.

- **Nutrition is Key:** Your stomach's got less room, but your body's need for nutrients hasn't shrunk. Keep vitamin and mineral supplements on hand to ensure you're getting all the good stuff your body craves for healing.

- **Knowledge is Power:** Don't let the 'what-ifs' scare you. Dive into the experiences of others who've walked this path and arm yourself with knowledge. Support groups and forums aren't just for learning—they're your cheer squad as you recover.

- **Kick the Habits:** If you smoke, consider surgery your cue to quit. Smoking's a recovery slow-down and a health hazard. And alcohol? Not the best idea when you're healing, especially with a tender throat post-intubation.

- **Pain Management Post-Pills:** Once the prescription painkillers are gone, you'll want something to tackle any lingering aches. Keep some over-the-counter options in your medicine cabinet for those just-in-case moments.

- **Comfort is King:** Waking up post-surgery, you'll want nothing to do with tight-fitting fashion. Loose, soft clothes are your best friends, especially ones that won't irritate your stitches. Keep it comfy at home and opt for relaxed fits at work until you're fully healed.

In the next few chapters, we will explore the different stages of recovery after your gastric sleeve surgery and the various recipes suitable for every stage of your recovery. Stay tuned as we explore the treasure trove of the bariatric diet.

Chapter 2

Phase 1: The Clear Liquids Diet

Hey there, fellow navigator of change! As you embark on this incredible transformation, Phase 1 is your first port of call. It's like the gentle morning dew, pure and simple. In this phase, we're focusing on clear liquids. But what does that mean for you? Let's break it down.

Imagine your stomach as a delicate new ecosystem, fresh and sensitive. We want to introduce it to the world slowly and gently. So, for the first 7 days post-surgery, you'll be sipping on liquids clearer than a crystal stream. We're talking about water that's as pristine as the sky on a sunny day, broths that are as comforting as a warm blanket, and sugar-free gelatin that's as light as a cloud.

But it's not just about what you drink; it's about how you drink it. Picture yourself savoring each sip, letting your body absorb every drop with gratitude. It's a time to be mindful, to be present, and to listen to the subtle cues your body gives you.

And let's not forget about hydration. It's the cornerstone of this phase. Your body is healing, and like a plant needs water to grow, you need these fluids to recover. They're not just filling your stomach; they're nourishing your soul, hydrating your cells, and flushing out the old to make way for the new.

Now, you might be wondering about variety. Fear not! There's a symphony of clear liquids out there. From the tang of a sugar-free popsicle to the warmth of a caffeine-free herbal tea, each one plays its part in your recovery. And if you're craving a hint of flavor, sugar-free flavored waters can add a splash of excitement to your liquid lineup.

As you glide through Phase 1, remember, this is just the beginning. Each clear liquid is a ripple in the pond of your new life, a life where health and happiness are in sync. So, take it slow, embrace the clarity, and let's toast (with water, of course) to your health and the journey ahead.

Hydrating Clear Broth

In the initial phase after bariatric surgery, it's crucial to stay hydrated and consume nutrients without solid foods. This Hydrating Clear Broth is perfect as it is gentle on the stomach, easy to digest, and provides essential electrolytes to help with hydration.

Ingredients

- 4 cups of water
- 2 chicken or vegetable bouillon cubes (ensure they are sugar-free and low-sodium)
- 1 teaspoon of salt (optional, based on dietary restrictions and doctor's advice)
- Herbs for flavor (such as thyme and parsley, tied together for easy removal)

Preparation Instructions

- In a medium-sized pot, bring the water to a boil.

- Add the bouillon cubes to the boiling water and stir until completely dissolved.
- Add the bundle of herbs for flavor.
- Reduce heat and let simmer for 10-15 minutes to infuse the broth with the herbs' flavors.
- Remove the pot from heat and discard the herbs.
- Allow the broth to cool to a comfortable temperature before serving.

Nutritional Value

This broth is designed to be light on the stomach and does not contribute significant calories or macronutrients. Its primary purpose is hydration and electrolyte balance.

Nutritional Information

- Calories: 5-10 per cup (varies based on the specific bouillon cubes used)
- Protein: 0-1g
- Carbohydrates: 1-2g
- Fat: 0g
- Sugar: 0g

<u>**Expert Tips**</u>

- Ensure the bouillon cubes used are appropriate for a clear liquid diet and do not contain any solid bits or high amounts of sodium.

- Feel free to experiment with different herbs to find a flavor profile that is soothing and enjoyable.

- Always check with your dietitian or surgeon before adding anything new to your post-op diet to ensure it is safe and appropriate for your current stage of recovery.

<u>**Cooking Time**</u>

20 minutes (including preparation and simmering time)

Sugar-Free Gelatin Dessert

The first phase after bariatric surgery emphasizes the importance of liquids and minimizing intake of sugars and solid foods. This Sugar-Free Gelatin Dessert is an excellent choice for patients transitioning through this phase. It's gentle on the stomach, helps with hydration, and adds a touch of variety in flavor without introducing sugars or fats.

Ingredients

- 1 packet of sugar-free gelatin powder (any flavor)
- 1 cup boiling water
- 1 cup cold water

Preparation Instructions

- In a heatproof bowl, dissolve the sugar-free gelatin powder in 1 cup of boiling water. Stir continuously until the gelatin is completely dissolved.
- Add 1 cup of cold water to the mixture and stir well.

- Pour the gelatin mixture into a shallow dish or individual serving cups.

- Refrigerate for at least 2 hours, or until the gelatin is firm and fully set.

- Serve chilled. If desired, cut into small, bite-sized pieces that are easier to consume.

Nutritional Value

This Sugar-Free Gelatin Dessert is crafted to be light and suitable for the post-surgical diet, focusing on hydration and avoiding sugars and solid food intake during the initial recovery phase.

Nutritional Information

- Calories: Approx. 10-20 per serving, depending on the brand of sugar-free gelatin
- Protein: 1-2g
- Carbohydrates: 0-1g
- Fat: 0g
- Sugar: 0g

Expert Tips

- Choosing a variety of flavors can help keep your diet interesting and make it easier to stay on track with your fluid intake.

- Ensure the gelatin is completely dissolved in boiling water to achieve the right consistency once it sets.

- For an added twist, consider adding a splash of decaffeinated herbal tea to the cold water portion for extra flavor. Ensure this is approved by your healthcare provider.

Cooking Time

Preparation time is about 5 minutes, with an additional 2 hours required for chilling and setting in the refrigerator.

Lemon-Lime Electrolyte Ice Pops

During Phase 1 of the bariatric diet, maintaining hydration and electrolyte balance is paramount. These Lemon-Lime Electrolyte Ice Pops are not only refreshing but also provide a boost of electrolytes, essential for patients recovering from surgery. They offer a flavorful way to stay hydrated and can be a pleasant diversion from plain water or other clear liquids.

Ingredients

- 2 cups of sugar-free electrolyte water (lemon-lime flavored)
- Juice of 1 fresh lemon
- Juice of 1 fresh lime
- Ice pop molds or small paper cups and popsicle sticks

Preparation Instructions

- In a pitcher, mix the lemon-lime flavored electrolyte water with the freshly squeezed lemon and lime juice.
- Pour the mixture into ice pop molds or small paper cups. If using paper cups, cover the top with plastic wrap and insert a popsicle stick through the center.
- Freeze for at least 4 hours or until solid.
- Once frozen, remove the ice pops from the molds or tear away the paper cups before serving.

Nutritional Value

These ice pops are designed to be low in calories while helping to replenish electrolytes lost during surgery or through limited food intake.

Nutritional Information

- Calories: Approx. 5-10 per ice pop (depending on the specific electrolyte water used)
- Protein: 0g

- Carbohydrates: 2-3g (primarily from the natural sugars in lemon and lime juice)
- Fat: 0g
- Sugar: 0-1g (natural sugars from the fruit)

Expert Tips

- Ensure the electrolyte water chosen is sugar-free and suitable for a clear liquid diet phase.
- Adjust the amount of lemon and lime juice to taste. More juice will result in a stronger, tangier flavor.
- For a smoother removal from molds, briefly run warm water over the outside of the molds before pulling the pops out.

Cooking Time

About 5 minutes to prepare, with a minimum of 4 hours to freeze until solid.

Clear Apple Juice Sipper

Staying hydrated and gently introducing flavors back into the diet is crucial in the first phase post-bariatric surgery. The Clear Apple Juice Sipper is a light, refreshing beverage designed for this very purpose. Made with diluted clear apple juice, it's easy on the stomach, providing hydration along with a subtle taste of sweetness from the apple. This drink is ideal for those looking to vary their liquid intake while adhering to the guidelines of Phase 1 of the bariatric diet.

Ingredients

- 1 cup of clear apple juice (ensure it's sugar-free and without pulp)
- 1 cup of water (for dilution)
- Ice cubes (optional, for serving)

Preparation Instructions

- In a large glass or pitcher, combine the clear apple juice with an equal amount of water to dilute the juice, making it lighter and more suitable for the clear liquid diet phase.

- Stir well to ensure the mixture is evenly diluted.
- Serve chilled, with or without ice cubes, according to preference.

Nutritional Value

This sipper provides a way to hydrate while introducing a mild flavor to the diet. It's intentionally light, aligning with the dietary restrictions of the early post-operative period.

Nutritional Information

- Calories: Approx Approx. 60-70 per serving, given the dilution (this can vary based on the specific apple juice brand used)
- Protein: 0g
- Carbohydrates: 15-17g (primarily from natural sugars in the apple juice, halved due to dilution)
- Fat: 0g
- Sugar: 15-17g (natural sugars from the apple, reduced due to dilution)

<u>**Expert Tips**</u>

- Always choose a clear apple juice that is free from pulp and added sugars to ensure it complies with the clear liquid diet requirements.

- Adjust the dilution to your taste and tolerance, especially in the early stages post-surgery when your stomach is most sensitive.

- Keeping this sipper chilled can provide a more refreshing experience, especially beneficial for hydration on warmer days.

<u>**Cooking Time**</u>

5 minutes or less to prepare, with additional chilling time if preferred.

Herbal Tea Infusion

In the immediate aftermath of bariatric surgery, maintaining adequate hydration is key, yet it's also important to introduce some variety to avoid monotony. Herbal Tea Infusion is an excellent choice for this phase, offering a soothing, flavorful alternative to plain water. Free from caffeine and gentle on the stomach, herbal teas can provide a comforting warmth or refreshing coolness, depending on how they're served.

Ingredients

- 1 herbal tea bag (choose a flavor that is caffeine-free and appealing, such as peppermint, chamomile, or hibiscus)
- 1 cup boiling water
- Ice cubes (optional, for serving cold)

Preparation Instructions

- Place the herbal tea bag in a large, heatproof cup.
- Pour 1 cup of boiling water over the tea bag.

- Allow the tea to steep for 3-5 minutes, depending on your taste preference for strength.

- Remove the tea bag and allow the tea to cool to a comfortable drinking temperature. For a cold beverage, allow the tea to come to room temperature before adding ice cubes to chill.

Nutritional Value

Herbal tea is naturally low in calories and free from sugar, making it an ideal choice for post-surgery hydration. It also offers the added benefit of potentially aiding digestion and reducing inflammation, depending on the herbs used.

Nutritional Information

- Calories: Approx. 0-5 per serving
- Protein: 0g
- Carbohydrates: 0-1g
- Fat:
- Sugar: 0g

Expert Tips

- Explore a variety of herbal tea flavors to keep your hydration routine interesting. Many herbal teas offer their own unique health benefits, such as chamomile for relaxation or peppermint for digestion.
- Always check that the tea is caffeine-free and avoid teas with added sugars or artificial flavors to ensure it complies with the clear liquid diet phase requirements.
- Herbal teas can be enjoyed warm or cold, making them versatile. In the early stages of recovery, test both temperature options to see what is most soothing for you.

Cooking Time

Less than 5 minutes to prepare, plus additional time for cooling or chilling if desired.

Cranberry Juice Splash

Hydration is a cornerstone of the post-bariatric surgery recovery process, especially during Phase 1, which focuses on clear liquids. The Cranberry Juice Splash offers a flavorful, refreshing option that's both hydrating and palatable, providing a nice change from water and herbal teas.

Ingredients

- 1 cup sugar-free cranberry juice (ensure it's clear and without pulp)
- 1 cup water (for dilution)
- Ice cubes (optional, for serving)

Preparation Instructions

- In a pitcher or large glass, mix the sugar-free cranberry juice with an equal part of water to dilute the juice. This makes the drink lighter and more appropriate for the clear liquid diet phase.

- Stir the mixture well to ensure it's evenly mixed.

- Serve the Cranberry Juice Splash chilled, adding ice cubes if desired for an extra refreshing experience.

Nutritional Value

Diluting the cranberry juice not only makes this drink suitable for the clear liquid phase but also lowers the concentration of natural sugars, making it a low-calorie option that's easy on the newly operated stomach.

Nutritional Information

- Calories: Approx. Approximately 15-30 per serving, depending on the cranberry juice brand
- Protein: 0g
- Carbohydrates: 3-5g (mostly from natural fruit sugars, reduced due to dilution)
- Fat: 0g
- Sugar: 2-4g (natural sugars, lower due to the dilution)

<u>**Expert Tips**</u>

- Look for cranberry juice that is labeled "clear" and "sugar-free" to comply with the clear liquid diet requirements and to avoid unnecessary sugars.

- Adjust the amount of water for dilution based on personal preference and tolerance, especially as the digestive system may be sensitive post-surgery.

- Cranberry juice is known for its urinary tract health benefits. However, always consult with your healthcare provider before adding anything new to your post-surgery diet to ensure it's safe for you.

<u>**Cooking Time**</u>

Less than 5 minutes to prepare, with no cooking required, just chilling if preferred.

Clear Chicken Consommé

Fresh out of surgery? Your tummy probably needs some TLC. Our Clear Chicken Consommé is a perfect pick for this stage. It's packed with protein and flavor, but gentle enough for your tummy. Think of it as a warm hug in a cup! This consommé is super clear because we've taken out all the greasy bits, making it ideal for Phase 1 of your bariatric journey.

Ingredients

- 4 cups of low-sodium chicken broth
- 1 egg white (used to clarify the broth, then removed)
- 1 small carrot, finely chopped (optional, for flavor, removed after cooking)
- 1 small celery stalk, finely chopped (optional, for flavor, removed after cooking)
- 1 sprig of fresh thyme (optional, for flavor, removed after cooking)

Preparation Instructions

- In a large pot, bring the chicken broth to a gentle simmer over medium heat.

- If using, add the carrot, celery, and thyme to the pot for added flavor. Let these simmer for about 20 minutes.

- In a small bowl, whisk the egg white lightly until frothy.

- Slowly pour the whisked egg white into the simmering broth. The egg white will attract and trap any solids and fats, clarifying the broth.

- Continue to simmer for another 10 minutes, then remove the pot from the heat.

- Strain the consommé through a fine-mesh sieve or cheesecloth into another pot or large bowl, ensuring no solids are left in the liquid.

- Serve the consommé warm, or let it cool and refrigerate for a chilled version.

Nutritional Value

This Clear Chicken Consommé is designed to be low in calories and fats, making it an excellent hydration source that also offers the soothing flavors and nutritional benefits of chicken broth.

Nutritional Information

- Calories: Approx. 5-10 per cup
- Protein: 1-2g
- Carbohydrates: 1-2g
- Fat: 0g
- Sugar: 0g

Expert Tips

The addition of egg white for clarification is a classic technique in making consommé, but it's essential to strain the broth thoroughly afterward to ensure it remains clear and suitable for a liquid diet.

Cooking Time

About 5 minutes to prepare, with a minimum of 4 hours to freeze until solid.

Sugar-Free Lemonade

Staying hydrated after surgery can feel like a chore, right? But it's super important! That's where our Sugar-Free Lemonade comes in. It's like a cool, refreshing hug for your taste buds, perfect for when water just won't cut it. Plus, it's sugar-free, so it fits perfectly with your post-surgery diet. No added sugar, but all the yummy tangy taste you know and love. It'll help you stay hydrated and happy during your recovery!

Ingredients

- 1 cup freshly squeezed lemon juice (about 4-6 lemons, depending on size and juiciness)
- 4 cups water
- Sugar substitute equivalent to 1 cup sugar (use a bariatric-friendly option such as stevia, erythritol, or monk fruit sweetener)
- Ice cubes (optional, for serving)

Preparation Instructions

- In a large pitcher, combine the freshly squeezed lemon juice with the water.

- Add the sugar substitute to the lemon and water mixture. Stir well until the sweetener is fully dissolved.

- Taste and adjust the sweetness if necessary, adding more sweetener to your preference.

- Chill in the refrigerator for at least 1 hour, or serve immediately over ice cubes for a refreshing drink.

Nutritional Value

This Sugar-Free Lemonade is a great way to keep hydrated and enjoy a sweet treat without adding sugar to your diet. It's especially beneficial during the early post-operative diet to avoid dehydration.

Nutritional Information

- Calories: 5-10 per serving (mainly from the lemon juice)
- Protein: 0g

- Carbohydrates: 2-3g 2-3g (from the natural sugars in lemon juice)
- Fat: 0g
- Sugar: 0g (no added sugars; contains natural sugars from lemons)

Expert Tips

- Ensure that the sugar substitute you choose is suitable for a clear liquid diet and is well-tolerated by your digestive system post-surgery.
- Freshly squeezed lemon juice is recommended for the best flavor and nutritional value, but ensure no pulp ends up in the lemonade to keep it clear.

Cooking Time

Less than 10 minutes to prepare, plus chilling time if preferred cold.

Broth-Infused Ice Chips

Staying hydrated after surgery is key, but plain water can get a bit boring, right? We hear you! That's where our Broth-Infused Ice Chips come in. They're like little flavor bombs for your mouth, made with yummy broth instead of plain water. Plus, they have some special stuff in them called electrolytes, which are super important for your body. They'll help you stay hydrated and feeling good while you recover.

Ingredients

- 2 cups of clear, low-sodium chicken or vegetable broth
- Ice cube trays or a shallow dish

Preparation Instructions

- Begin by heating the broth in a saucepan over medium heat until it's warm but not boiling. Heating the broth can help intensify its flavors.

- Carefully pour the warm broth into ice cube trays or a shallow dish. If using a shallow dish, you'll break the frozen layer into chips later.
- Place the trays or dish into the freezer. Freeze until solid, approximately 2-4 hours, depending on your freezer settings.
- Once frozen, if you've used a shallow dish, use a fork or the back of a spoon to gently break the layer into small, chip-sized pieces.
- Store the ice chips in a freezer-safe container or bag for easy access.

Nutritional Value

Broth-Infused Ice Chips offer the hydrating benefits of clear liquids while providing the added bonus of electrolytes and a slight protein boost from the broth, making them a nutrient-rich alternative to plain ice chips.

Nutritional Information

- Calories: Approximately 5-10 per serving (depending on the type of broth used)
- Protein: 1-2g
- Carbohydrates: 0-1g
- Fat: 0g
- Sugar: 0g

Expert Tips

- Choose a broth that is flavorful yet clear, as cloudiness can indicate higher fat content or solid particles, which should be avoided during the clear liquid phase.

- Experiment with different types of broth for variety. Beef, chicken, and vegetable broths each offer a unique flavor profile.

- If you're sensitive to cold temperatures, let the ice chips slightly soften at room temperature for a few moments before consuming them.

Cooking Time

Less than 5 minutes to prepare, plus 2-4 hours freezing time.

Peppermint Tea Cooler

Feeling a little queasy after surgery? Don't worry, we've got your back (and tummy!). Our Peppermint Tea Cooler is like a gentle hug for your insides. Peppermint tea is famous for calming things down, which can be a big help when you're healing. Plus, it's caffeine-free, so it fits perfectly with your post-surgery diet. This cooler is a fun twist on regular tea – think cool, minty refreshment to keep you hydrated and feeling your best!

Ingredients

- 2 peppermint tea bags
- 4 cups boiling water
- Ice cubes
- Optional: A few fresh peppermint leaves for garnish

<u>**Preparation Instructions**</u>

- Steep the peppermint tea bags in the boiling water for 5-7 minutes, depending on your preferred strength.

- Remove the tea bags and allow the tea to cool to room temperature.

- Once cooled, pour the tea over a glass full of ice cubes to chill it quickly. Alternatively, refrigerate the tea until it's cold and serve over ice.

- If desired, add a few fresh peppermint leaves to the glass for a garnish and an extra burst of peppermint flavor.

<u>**Nutritional Value**</u>

This Peppermint Tea Cooler is practically calorie-free and provides a soothing, hydrating beverage option that fits perfectly within the clear liquid diet requirements. Peppermint itself has been noted for its digestive benefits, which can be particularly helpful during post-surgery recovery.

Nutritional Information

- Calories: Approx. 0-5 per serving
- Protein: 0g
- Carbohydrates: 0-1g
- Fat: 0g
- Sugar: 0g

Expert Tips

- Ensure the tea is fully cooled before serving to avoid any potential discomfort from consuming warm liquids too quickly post-surgery.
- For those later in their recovery process, experimenting with blending peppermint tea with other approved clear liquids for new flavor combinations can keep your hydration routine interesting.

Cooking Time

Preparation takes about 10 minutes, with additional cooling time as needed.

Chapter 3

Phase 2: The Protein-Based Liquids Diet

Alright, let's roll up our sleeves and dive into Phase 2 of your bariatric diet, where things start getting a little more interesting. This is the stage where we introduce a bit more substance to your meals, but we're still keeping things smooth and easy to digest.

Think of Phase 2 as the 'thick liquid' stage. It's like the transition from a clear morning sky to a day filled with fluffy clouds. We're moving on from the crystal-clear liquids of Phase 1 to the more satisfying, protein-packed liquids that'll make your taste buds dance and your muscles thank you.

During this phase, which typically spans from the end of week 1 to about week 4 post-surgery, you'll be savoring things like creamy protein shakes, silky smooth soups, and even some pureed foods if your doctor gives the thumbs up.

It's all about giving your body the nutrients it needs to heal without putting too much strain on your tender tummy.

Now, let's talk portions. Remember, your stomach is still the size of a tiny pouch, so we're not hosting a feast here. You'll likely feel full after just a few spoonfuls, and that's perfectly okay. It's essential to listen to your body and let it guide you. A couple of tablespoons here, a quarter cup there, and you're on your way to a happy, satisfied stomach.

And here's a pro tip: establish a mealtime routine. Set specific times for your meals and stick to them. It's like setting regular coffee dates with your stomach, and trust me, it loves punctuality.

So, what's on the menu for Phase 2? We've got a lineup of stars ready to nourish you:

- **Protein Shakes:** These are your new best friends, packed with the protein your body craves.
- **Blended Soups:** Imagine the comforting embrace of a warm, blended soup. Go for varieties like lentil, black bean, or split pea.

- **Pureed Fruits and Veggies:** Soft, pureed fruits and veggies are like a gentle pat on the back for your digestive system.

- **Cottage Cheese:** It's soft, it's creamy, and it's oh-so-protein-rich.

- **Yogurt:** Plain or Greek, it's a smooth operator that'll keep you and your stomach in harmony.

As you navigate through Phase 2, remember to take it slow. Savor each spoonful, enjoy the new flavors, and celebrate the small victories. Your journey is unique, and every step forward is a step towards a healthier you. So, here's to thick liquids and the smooth road to recovery!"

Creamy Vanilla Protein Shake

Phase 2 of your bariatric journey just got a whole lot yummier! This shake is like a party in your mouth – creamy banana meets delicious peanut butter, all blended together with a protein boost that helps your body heal strong. Think of it as a tasty reward for all your hard work!

Ingredients

- 1 scoop of high-quality vanilla whey protein isolate powder
- 1 cup unsweetened almond milk (or any preferred milk alternative)
- Ice cubes, as desired for thickness
- ¼ teaspoon vanilla extract (for an extra flavor boost)
- Optional: A pinch of cinnamon or nutmeg for garnish

Preparation Instructions

- In a blender, combine the vanilla whey protein isolate, unsweetened almond milk, and vanilla extract.
- Add ice cubes to achieve the desired thickness of your shake.
- Blend on high until the mixture is smooth and creamy.
- Pour the shake into a glass and, if desired, sprinkle a pinch of cinnamon or nutmeg on top for garnish

Nutritional Value

This shake is specifically formulated to support your protein needs post-surgery, offering a significant amount of high-quality protein to aid in recovery and muscle maintenance during the liquid phase of your diet.

Nutritional Information

- Calories: Approximately 150-200 (varies by protein powder brand and type of milk used)
- Protein: 20-25g
- Carbohydrates: 3-8g

- Fat: 2-5g
- Sugar: 1-3g

Expert Tips

- Ensure the protein powder you select is low in sugar and high in protein, ideally whey protein isolate for its high digestibility and purity.

- If you're lactose intolerant or prefer a dairy-free option, ensure both the protein powder and the milk alternative suit your dietary needs.

- The addition of ice not only chills the shake but also adds to its creamy texture, making it more satisfying to drink.

Cooking Time

Less than 5 minutes to prepare.

The Creamy Vanilla Protein Shake is a cornerstone recipe for anyone in Phase 2 of the bariatric diet, blending essential nutrition with enjoyable flavors. It's a simple, quick way to meet your protein requirements while keeping your palate satisfied.

Chicken Bone Broth Protein Soup

Phase 2 is all about leveling up your recovery game, and this shake is your secret weapon! It's a flavor explosion with creamy banana and rich peanut butter, but don't forget the hidden superpower: protein! It helps your body heal and build strong muscles, so you can conquer this phase with a smile (and a full tummy).

Ingredients

- 4 cups of homemade or store-bought chicken bone broth (ensure it's low-sodium and without additives)
- 1 scoop of unflavored protein powder (whey or collagen-based for easy digestion)
- Salt and pepper to taste
- Optional: Fresh herbs like parsley or thyme for flavor

<u>**Preparation Instructions**</u>

- In a medium saucepan, gently heat the chicken bone broth over low to medium heat. Avoid boiling to preserve the nutrients.

- Once the broth is warm, slowly whisk in the scoop of unflavored protein powder until fully dissolved and the mixture is smooth.

- Season the soup with a pinch of salt and pepper to taste. Remember, your taste preferences may be different post-surgery, so start with smaller amounts and adjust as needed.

- If using, add a few fresh herbs for additional flavor. Let them simmer in the soup for a few minutes, then remove before serving.

- Serve the soup warm, ensuring it's not too hot for consumption.

<u>**Nutritional Value**</u>

This soup leverages the nutritional powerhouse of chicken bone broth, renowned for its collagen, minerals, and amino acids, with added protein to support tissue repair and muscle maintenance during the recovery phase.

<u>**Nutritional Information**</u>

- Calories: Approximately 100-150 per serving,
- Protein: 20-30g
- Carbohydrates: 1-2g
- Fat: 1-2g
- Sugar: 0g

<u>**Expert Tips**</u>

Introducing protein powder to the warm broth requires careful whisking to avoid clumping. A blender can also be used to ensure smoothness.

<u>**Cooking Time**</u>

About 10 minutes to warm the broth and dissolve the protein powder.

The Chicken Bone Broth Protein Soup is a foundational recipe for those in Phase 2 of the bariatric recovery diet. Its warm, soothing nature, combined with a protein boost, makes it an ideal choice for those seeking comfort and nourishment while adhering to the dietary guidelines necessary for a successful recovery.

High-Protein Beef Broth Smoothie

This High-Protein Beef Broth Smoothie might sound a little different, but trust us, it's amazing. We've taken savory beef broth and blended it with a protein boost, making a delicious umami-packed drink that's way more exciting than plain broth. Think of it as a warm hug for your tummy, packed with all the good stuff to help you conquer this next step!"

Ingredients

- 2 cups of high-quality, low-sodium beef bone broth, heated
- 1 scoop of unflavored or beef-flavored protein powder (collagen or whey-based)
- A pinch of sea salt (optional, to taste)
- A pinch of ground black pepper (optional, to taste)
- Optional for enhanced flavor: a dash of Worcestershire sauce or herbs like rosemary or thyme

<u>**Preparation Instructions**</u>

- Warm the beef bone broth in a saucepan over medium heat until it's hot but not boiling.

- Transfer the warm broth to a blender. Add the scoop of protein powder, and if using, the Worcestershire sauce or herbs.

- Blend on a low speed at first, gradually increasing to ensure the mixture is thoroughly combined and smooth.

- Taste and season with a pinch of sea salt and ground black pepper if desired.

- Serve the smoothie warm, like a sipping broth, or allow it to cool and consume it chilled, based on personal preference.

<u>**Nutritional Value**</u>

This savory smoothie is an excellent source of protein and collagen, derived from the beef broth and supplemental protein powder, supporting tissue repair and muscle maintenance during post-surgery recovery.

Nutritional Information

- Calories: Approximately 100-200, depending on the protein powder used
- Protein: 20-30g
- Carbohydrates: 1-3g
- Fat: 0.5-2g
- Sugar: 0g

Expert Tips

- Choose a high-quality beef bone broth for the best nutritional content and flavor.
- If the concept of a savory smoothie is new to you, start with a small batch to adjust the flavors to your liking.

Cooking Time

About 5 minutes for heating the broth and additional time for blending.

This High-Protein Beef Broth Smoothie offers a novel way to incorporate more protein into the diet during the critical recovery phase following bariatric surgery. Its savory profile provides a welcome alternative for those seeking variety beyond traditional sweet protein shakes.

Greek Yogurt and Berry Protein Smoothie

Missing some sweetness in Phase 2? We've got you covered! This Greek Yogurt and Berry Protein Smoothie is like a creamy dream come true. We've blended yummy Greek yogurt with a burst of antioxidant-rich berries, all packed with a protein punch. It's the perfect way to satisfy your sweet tooth while keeping your protein goals on track.

Ingredients

- 1 cup plain, low-fat Greek yogurt
- ½ cup mixed berries (such as strawberries, blueberries, raspberries), fresh or frozen
- ½ cup water or unsweetened almond milk to thin the smoothie
- 1 scoop of vanilla or unflavored protein powder
- Ice cubes (optional, for desired consistency)

Preparation Instructions

- Place the Greek yogurt, mixed berries, and protein powder in a blender.
- Add water or almond milk to help blend the ingredients smoothly. Adjust the amount to reach your preferred consistency.
- Blend on high until the mixture is smooth and creamy. If the smoothie is too thick, you can add a little more liquid to thin it out.
- For a colder smoothie, add a few ice cubes to the blender and blend until smooth.
- Pour the smoothie into a glass and enjoy immediately.

Nutritional Value

This smoothie is packed with high-quality protein from both Greek yogurt and protein powder, vital for muscle repair and growth post-surgery. The berries add dietary fiber, vitamins, and antioxidants, making this beverage as nutritious as it is delicious.

Nutritional Information

- Calories: Approximately 200-300
- Protein: 20-40g (depending on the brand and amount of Greek yogurt and protein powder used)
- Carbohydrates: 15-30g
- Fat: 0-5g
- Sugar: Naturally occurring sugars from the berries and yogurt

Expert Tips

- If you're using frozen berries, there's no need to add ice unless you prefer an extra-thick smoothie.
- For those watching their sugar intake closely, be sure to select a protein powder that is low in sugar and carbohydrates.

Cooking Time

5 minutes

The Greek Yogurt and Berry Protein Smoothie offers a delightful and easy way to meet your protein requirements during Phase 2 of the bariatric diet. Its combination of flavors not only makes for a refreshing meal replacement or snack but also provides essential nutrients to aid in your recovery and health maintenance.

Savory Pumpkin Protein Soup

Feeling a little chilly after surgery? This Savory Pumpkin Protein Soup is like a warm hug in a bowl! We've blended creamy pumpkin with a protein boost to create a delicious and nutritious soup. It's packed with vitamins and minerals, making it the perfect comfort food for this phase of your journey. Plus, it's full of protein, which is just what your body needs to heal strong!

Ingredients

- 2 cups pure pumpkin puree (ensure it's 100% pumpkin, with no added sugars or spices)
- 2 cups low-sodium vegetable broth or chicken broth
- 1 scoop unflavored protein powder (whey or plant-based for easy digestion)
- ½ teaspoon ground cinnamon
- ¼ teaspoon ground nutmeg
- Salt and pepper to taste
- Optional: a dash of ground ginger for extra warmth

<u>**Preparation Instructions**</u>

- In a medium saucepan, combine the pumpkin puree and broth. Stir well to mix.

- Warm the mixture over medium heat, stirring occasionally, until it begins to simmer gently.

- Reduce the heat to low. Whisk in the protein powder thoroughly until no lumps remain.

- Season the soup with cinnamon, nutmeg, and, if using, ginger. Add salt and pepper to your taste.

- Continue to simmer the soup for another 5-10 minutes, allowing the flavors to meld together.

- Taste and adjust the seasoning as necessary before removing from heat.

- Serve the soup warm, or let it cool and gently reheat before serving if prepared in advance.

<u>**Nutritional Value**</u>

This soup combines the health benefits of pumpkin, such as fiber, potassium, and beta-carotene, with the muscle-repairing and building benefits of protein powder, creating a well-rounded meal that supports recovery.

Nutritional Information

- Calories: Approximately 150-200 per serving
- Protein: 15-25g
- Carbohydrates: 10-20g
- Fat: 0-2g
- Sugar: Low, depending on the natural sugars in the pumpkin puree

Expert Tips

The protein powder should be unflavored to maintain the savory profile of the soup; however, ensure it dissolves completely to avoid altering the soup's texture.

Cooking Time

15-20 minutes

Savory Pumpkin Protein Soup is an excellent addition to the diet in Phase 2 of post-bariatric surgery recovery, offering a comforting and nutritious meal option. Its ease of preparation and rich flavor profile make it a welcome variation from typical protein shakes, supporting your journey towards recovery and health.

Egg White and Spinach Protein Soup

Phase 2 is all about protein power, and this Egg White and Spinach Protein Soup is a champion! We've blended fluffy egg whites with a powerhouse of vitamins from spinach, all in a delicious, easy-to-digest soup. It's like a healthy green smoothie in bowl form, packing a protein punch and keeping your tummy happy.

Ingredients

- 4 cups low-sodium chicken or vegetable broth
- 1 cup fresh spinach leaves, finely chopped
- 4 egg whites
- Salt and pepper to taste
- A pinch of nutmeg (optional, for added flavor)
- Optional: Fresh herbs like parsley or chives for garnish

Preparation Instructions

- In a medium saucepan, bring the broth to a simmer over medium heat.
- Add the chopped spinach to the broth and let it cook for 2-3 minutes until the spinach is wilted and bright green.
- In a bowl, lightly beat the egg whites until frothy. Slowly pour the beaten egg whites into the simmering broth, stirring gently with a fork to form thin strands of egg whites.
- Season the soup with salt, pepper, and a pinch of nutmeg if using. Continue to simmer for an additional 3-4 minutes, allowing the egg whites to cook through and the flavors to meld.
- Taste and adjust the seasoning as needed.
- Serve the soup hot, garnished with fresh herbs if desired.

Nutritional Value

This soup is an excellent source of lean protein from the egg whites, which are crucial for muscle repair and growth during recovery. Spinach adds fiber, iron, and vitamins A and C, contributing to the overall nutritional density of the meal.

Nutritional Information

- Calories: Approximately 100-150 per serving
- Protein: 15-20g
- Carbohydrates: 2-4g
- Fat: 0-1g
- Sugar: 0-1g

Expert Tips

Ensure the broth is kept at a gentle simmer when adding the egg whites to prevent them from curdling

Cooking Time

About 15 minutes

Egg White and Spinach Protein Soup is a comforting, nutritious option for those in Phase 2 of the bariatric diet, providing a delicious way to meet protein requirements while also incorporating vegetables into your diet.

Peanut Butter Chocolate Protein Shake

This Peanut Butter Chocolate Protein Shake is like a guilt-free party in your mouth. We've blended creamy peanut butter with delicious chocolate, but don't forget the hidden hero: protein! It helps your body heal strong and keeps you feeling full, making this shake a perfect snack or even a meal replacement during Phase 2.

Ingredients

- 1 scoop of chocolate protein powder (whey or plant-based)
- 1 tablespoon natural, unsweetened peanut butter
- 1 cup unsweetened almond milk or other milk alternative
- Ice cubes, as needed for thickness
- Optional: a pinch of stevia or monk fruit sweetener for extra sweetness

<u>**Preparation Instructions**</u>

- In a blender, combine the chocolate protein powder, peanut butter, and almond milk.
- Add a few ice cubes to achieve your desired shake consistency.
- Blend on high until smooth and creamy.
- Taste and, if desired, add a pinch of stevia or monk fruit sweetener for additional sweetness. Blend again to incorporate.
- Pour the shake into a glass and enjoy immediately.

<u>**Nutritional Value**</u>

This shake is not only delicious but also packed with protein from the powder and healthy fats from the peanut butter, contributing to muscle repair and satiety. The addition of almond milk provides a low-calorie, dairy-free base that's gentle on the stomach.

<u>**Nutritional Information**</u>

- Calories: Approximately 200-300, depending on the protein powder and amount of peanut butter used
- Protein: 20-30g

- Carbohydrates: 5-15g
- Fat: 8-16g
- Sugar: 1-5g, largely depending on the protein powder used and if additional sweetener is added

Expert Tips

- Choosing a high-quality, low-sugar chocolate protein powder is crucial for maintaining the nutritional integrity of this shake.
- Natural, unsweetened peanut butter is recommended to avoid added sugars and oils.

Cooking Time

5 minutes

The Peanut Butter Chocolate Protein Shake is a delightful, easy-to-make option for those in Phase 2 of the bariatric diet. It offers a way to enjoy a treat-like experience without compromising your dietary goals, making it a perfect choice for a post-workout boost or a satisfying snack.

Almond Milk and Whey Protein Smoothie

This Almond Milk and Whey Protein Smoothie is your secret weapon. It's light, clean, and packed with high-quality protein to keep your body happy. We use yummy almond milk for a mild base and whey protein for a protein punch – no heavy flavors or weird additives here!

Ingredients

- 1 scoop of vanilla whey protein powder (or any flavor preferred)
- 1 cup unsweetened almond milk
- Ice cubes, as needed for desired consistency

Preparation Instructions

- Pour the almond milk into a blender.
- Add the scoop of whey protein powder.
- Add a few ice cubes to achieve the thickness you like in a smoothie.

- Blend on high until the mixture is smooth and the ice is fully incorporated.
- Taste and adjust—if the smoothie needs more sweetness, consider adding a pinch of stevia or monk fruit sweetener, then blend again.
- Serve immediately for the freshest flavor and best texture.

Nutritional Value

This smoothie focuses on providing a high protein intake with minimal additional ingredients, making it perfect for those needing a protein supplement without extra calories or sugars. Almond milk offers a low-calorie, dairy-free base, while whey protein supplies essential amino acids necessary for muscle repair and growth.

Nutritional Information

- Calories: Approximately 150-200, depending on the protein powder brand
- Protein: 20-25g
- Carbohydrates: 1-3g
- Fat: 2-4g

- Sugar: 0-1g, varies by almond milk and protein powder used

Expert Tips

- Ensure the whey protein powder is of high quality and low in additives for the best health benefits.

- If using a flavored protein powder, select one that complements the mild taste of almond milk without overwhelming it.

- For a creamier texture, add more ice or even a tablespoon of Greek yogurt (if tolerable and approved for your current diet stage).

Cooking Time

5 minutes

The Almond Milk and Whey Protein Smoothie offers a straightforward, nutritious option for those in Phase 2 of the bariatric diet. Its simplicity makes it an excellent choice for a quick breakfast, post-exercise recovery drink, or a protein-rich snack between meals.

Cottage Cheese and Peach Protein Smoothie

This Cottage Cheese and Peach Protein Smoothie is a flavor explosion in a glass. We've blended creamy, protein-packed cottage cheese with juicy peaches for a touch of natural sweetness and vitamins. It's the perfect way to keep your protein intake on track while enjoying a refreshing, delicious drink. Think of it as a taste bud adventure that fuels your body – yum!

Ingredients

- ½ cup low-fat cottage cheese
- 1 cup frozen peach slices
- ½ cup unsweetened almond milk or water (for blending)
- 1 scoop vanilla protein powder (optional, for an extra protein boost)
- Ice cubes (optional, for desired consistency)
- Optional: A pinch of cinnamon or nutmeg for added flavor

<u>**Preparation Instructions**</u>

- Add the cottage cheese, frozen peach slices, almond milk (or water), and protein powder (if using) into a blender.

- Blend on high until the mixture is smooth. If the smoothie is too thick, you can add a bit more almond milk or water until you reach your desired consistency.

- Taste the smoothie and, if desired, add a pinch of cinnamon or nutmeg for extra flavor. Blend again briefly to mix.

- If you prefer a colder smoothie, add ice cubes and blend until smooth.

- Pour into a glass and enjoy immediately.

<u>**Nutritional Value**</u>

Cottage cheese is a fantastic source of casein protein, which is slow-digesting and can help keep you feeling full longer. Peaches add a natural sweetness and provide dietary fiber, vitamins A and C, and antioxidants. This smoothie is a balanced option for a meal replacement or snack, supporting muscle repair and providing energy.

Nutritional Information

- Calories: Approximately 200-300, depending on the use of protein powder and type of milk
- Protein: 20-30g
- Carbohydrates: 15-25g
- Fat: 2-5g
- Sugar: 10-15g (mostly natural sugars from the peaches)

Expert Tips

If you're not a fan of peach, this smoothie can be adapted with other frozen fruits like berries or mango for different flavors.

Cooking Time

5 minutes

The Cottage Cheese and Peach Protein Smoothie is a flavorful, nutritious addition to the diet in Phase 2 of post-bariatric surgery recovery. It combines high-quality protein with the natural sweetness of fruit, offering a delicious way to meet dietary protein requirements while enjoying a variety of flavors.

Tomato Basil Protein Soup

Craving some comfort food in Phase 2? This Tomato Basil Protein Soup is your new BFF! We've blended juicy tomatoes with fresh basil for that classic taste you love, and then snuck in some extra protein to help your body heal strong. It's a delicious and nutritious way to keep your tummy happy and your protein goals on track. Think warm hug in a bowl, with a protein punch!

Ingredients

- 2 cups low-sodium tomato juice or pureed tomatoes
- 1 scoop of unflavored protein powder (whey or plant-based)
- ¼ cup fresh basil leaves, finely chopped
- Salt and pepper to taste
- Optional: A pinch of garlic powder or Italian seasoning for extra flavor

<u>**Preparation Instructions**</u>

- In a medium saucepan, gently heat the tomato juice or pureed tomatoes over medium heat until simmering.
- Reduce the heat to low and slowly whisk in the protein powder until fully dissolved and the mixture is smooth.
- Add the chopped basil to the soup, and if using, include garlic powder or Italian seasoning for an enhanced flavor profile.
- Season with salt and pepper to taste. Allow the soup to simmer for another 5-10 minutes, letting the flavors meld together.
- Taste and adjust the seasoning as needed before removing from heat.
- Serve the soup warm, garnished with a few fresh basil leaves if desired.

<u>**Nutritional Value**</u>

Tomatoes are rich in vitamins C and K, potassium, and antioxidants, offering health benefits like improved heart health and reduced inflammation.

Nutritional Information

- Calories: Approximately 100-150 per serving
- Protein: 15-25g
- Carbohydrates: 10-15g
- Fat: 0-1g
- Sugar: 6-8g (natural sugars from tomatoes)

Expert Tips

Choose a high-quality, low-sodium tomato juice or pureed tomatoes to control the salt content and ensure the healthiest base for your soup.

Cooking Time

About 15-20 minutes

The Tomato Basil Protein Soup is a heartwarming, nutritious addition to the Phase 2 bariatric diet, combining classic flavors with a much-needed protein boost. Its simplicity and the comforting nature make it a perfect meal option for anyone looking to enjoy traditional tastes while adhering to dietary requirements post-surgery.

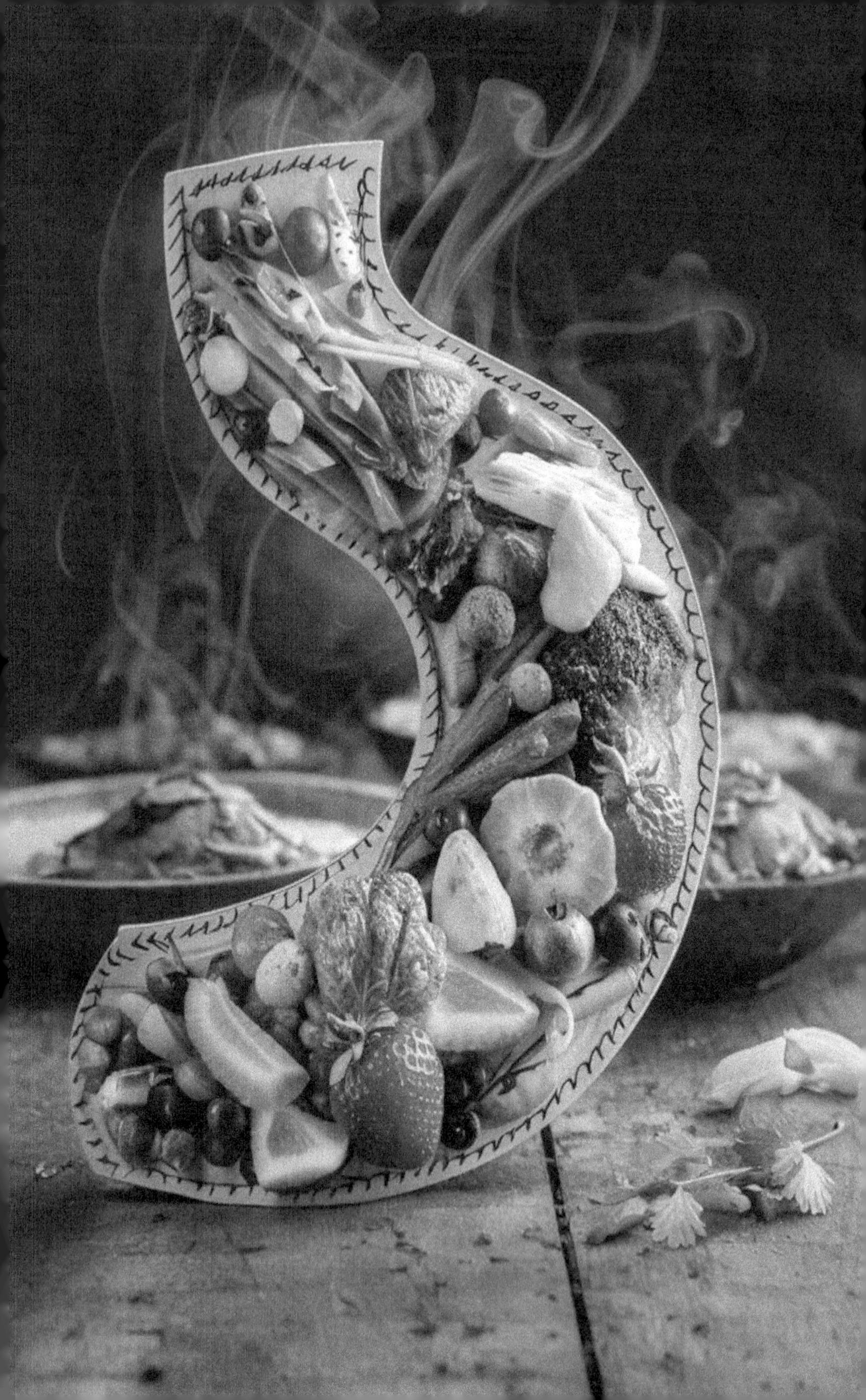

Chapter 4

Phase 3: The Pureed Foods Diet

Let's get cozy with Phase 3, the soft food fiesta! This is where your palate gets to play with a bit more texture, and your stomach gets to handle something a little heartier than liquids. It's like the soft jazz of the diet phases – smooth, mellow, and oh-so-satisfying.

Phase 3 usually kicks off around week 4 post-surgery and can last up to week 8. It's a time of culinary exploration within the soft food spectrum. We're talking about foods that are tender enough to be mashed with a fork, yet substantial enough to make your meals feel like... well, actual meals!

Here's the scoop: you'll be introducing a delightful array of proteins, veggies, and fruits into your diet. But we're not diving into a steak just yet. We're easing into it with foods like:

- **Eggs:** Scrambled, poached, or soft-boiled, they're your protein-packed buddies.

- **Cottage Cheese:** Creamy and versatile, it's a blank canvas for flavors.

- **Ripe Bananas:** Nature's own sweet treat, easy on the tummy and full of nutrients.

- **Avocado:** Smooth, rich, and full of healthy fats, it's like a hug for your heart.

- **Steamed Veggies:** Carrots, zucchini, and spinach, oh my! Soft, warm, and comforting.

And here's a golden rule for Phase 3: protein is still the star of the show. Start your meals with a bite of protein to keep those muscles strong and your recovery on track.

But wait, there's more! You're not just eating; you're relearning how to eat. Take small bites, chew thoroughly, and savor every morsel. It's not a race; it's a journey. And remember, if your stomach says 'stop,' you stop. No questions asked.

So, embrace the softness, enjoy the new tastes and textures, and celebrate every bite. Phase 3 is not just a phase; it's a milestone on your road to a healthier you. Cheers to soft foods and smoother days ahead!"

Avocado and Chicken Puree

Phase 3 is here, and it's time to level up your food game (gently)! This Avocado and Chicken Puree is like a flavor explosion for your tummy. We've blended creamy avocado with yummy chicken, packing it with healthy fats and protein to keep you feeling full and satisfied. Plus, it's super easy to digest, so your body can focus on healing strong.

Ingredients

- 1 small cooked chicken breast (boiled or poached, and then cooled)
- 1 ripe avocado
- A splash of low-sodium chicken broth or water (for adjusting consistency)
- Salt and pepper to taste
- Optional: A squeeze of lemon juice for added flavor

Preparation Instructions

- Ensure the chicken breast is cooked thoroughly, cooled, and has no skin or bones. Chop it into smaller pieces for easier blending.
- Scoop out the avocado flesh and add it to the blender with the chicken.
- Begin blending the chicken and avocado together, gradually adding a splash of chicken broth or water until you achieve a smooth, creamy consistency.
- Season the puree with salt and pepper to taste. If using, add a squeeze of lemon juice to enhance the flavors and add a bit of acidity.
- Blend again briefly to ensure all ingredients are fully combined.
- Taste and adjust the seasoning if necessary. The puree should be smooth and easy to eat with a spoon.

Nutritional Value

This puree offers a balanced mix of lean protein from the chicken and healthy fats from the avocado, along with a range of vitamins, minerals, and heart-healthy monounsaturated fats.

<u>**Nutritional Information**</u>

- Calories: Approximately 300-400 per serving
- Protein: 20-30g
- Carbohydrates: 9-15g
- Fat: 20-30g
- Sugar: 1-3g

<u>**Expert Tips**</u>

- For the best texture, use a ripe avocado that blends smoothly.

- Adding lemon juice not only boosts the flavor but also helps prevent the avocado from browning if you need to store the puree for a short period.

<u>**Cooking Time**</u>

Less than 10 minutes to prepare if the chicken is already cooked.

The Avocado and Chicken Puree is a nutritious, flavorful option for those progressing through Phase 3 of the bariatric diet. Its ease of preparation and balanced nutritional profile make it an excellent choice for a meal or substantial snack during this critical phase of recovery.

Broccoli and Cauliflower Cheese Puree

This Broccoli and Cauliflower Cheese Puree is a veggie fiesta in a bowl. We've blended healthy broccoli and cauliflower with creamy, delicious cheese to create a comforting and nutritious meal. It's gentle on your tummy but packed with fiber, vitamins, and protein – everything your body needs to keep thriving! Think of it as a warm hug on a plate, helping you conquer Phase 3 with a smile.

Ingredients

- 1 cup broccoli florets, steamed until very tender
- 1 cup cauliflower florets, steamed until very tender
- 1/4 cup low-fat cheddar cheese, shredded
- 2 tablespoons low-fat milk or unsweetened almond milk
- Salt and pepper to taste
- Optional: A pinch of garlic powder or nutmeg for added flavor

Preparation Instructions

- Steam the broccoli and cauliflower florets until they are very soft and easily pierced with a fork. Allow them to cool slightly.
- Place the steamed vegetables in a blender or food processor.
- Add the shredded low-fat cheddar cheese and milk to the blender. If desired, include garlic powder or nutmeg for extra flavor.
- Blend on high until the mixture reaches a smooth, creamy consistency. Add a little more milk if necessary to achieve the desired texture.
- Season the puree with salt and pepper to taste, then blend again briefly to mix.
- Serve warm, ensuring the cheese is fully melted and the puree is well combined.

Nutritional Value

This puree is an excellent way to enjoy the health benefits of broccoli and cauliflower, which are rich in dietary fiber, vitamins C and K, and antioxidants. The addition of low-fat cheddar cheese provides calcium and protein, making this meal both satisfying and nutritious.

<u>**Nutritional Information**</u>

- Calories: Approximately 150-200 per serving
- Protein: 10-15g
- Carbohydrates: 10-15g
- Fat: 5-10g
- Sugar: 3-5g

<u>**Expert Tips**</u>

- Ensure the vegetables are steamed to a very soft consistency to achieve a smooth puree suitable for Phase 3 of the bariatric diet.
- Adjust the amount of milk to achieve your preferred puree thickness. Some may prefer a thicker consistency, while others might like it slightly thinner.

<u>**Cooking Time**</u>

20-25 minutes

The Broccoli and Cauliflower Cheese Puree is a delightful, nutritious addition to the Phase 3 bariatric diet. Its creamy texture and comforting taste make it an appealing meal option, providing essential nutrients and protein in a form that's easy on the digestive system.

Cottage Cheese and Peach Puree

This Cottage Cheese and Peach Puree is like a taste bud party. We've blended creamy cottage cheese (protein power!) with juicy peaches for a burst of natural sweetness and vitamins. It's a delicious and satisfying option that keeps you feeling full and fueled throughout this phase.

Ingredients

- 1/2 cup low-fat cottage cheese
- 1 ripe peach, peeled and sliced (or equivalent canned peaches in natural juice, drained)
- A splash of milk or almond milk (if needed for blending)
- Optional: A pinch of cinnamon or vanilla extract for added flavor

Preparation Instructions

- If using a fresh peach, ensure it's ripe and sweet. Peel and slice the peach, removing the pit.
- In a blender, combine the low-fat cottage cheese and peach slices. If the peach is very ripe and juicy, you might not need additional liquid. If using canned peaches, ensure they are well-drained.
- Blend the mixture on high until completely smooth. If the puree is too thick, add a splash of milk or almond milk to reach your desired consistency.
- Taste the puree and, if desired, add a pinch of cinnamon or a few drops of vanilla extract for extra flavor. Blend again briefly to mix.
- Serve the puree chilled or at room temperature, depending on your preference.

Nutritional Value

This puree offers a great balance of protein from the cottage cheese, which is essential for healing and muscle maintenance, and carbohydrates from the peaches for energy. Additionally, peaches provide dietary fiber, vitamins, and minerals.

Nutritional Information

- Calories: Approximately 100-150 per serving Protein: 10-15g
- Carbohydrates: 10-20g
- Fat: 0.5-2g
- Sugar: 8-15g (natural sugars from the peaches)

Expert Tips

- Choose low-fat cottage cheese to keep the puree light and healthy.
- For a smoother texture, you can strain the puree through a sieve to remove any remaining lumps, although a good blender should make this unnecessary.

Cooking Time

10 minutes

The Cottage Cheese and Peach Puree is a delightful, easy-to-make addition to the Phase 3 bariatric diet. Its creamy, sweet profile makes it an enjoyable way to meet dietary protein needs while introducing the natural sweetness of fruit into your meals.

Creamy Spinach and White Bean Puree

This Creamy Spinach and White Bean Puree is a hidden champion. We've blended iron-packed spinach with protein and fiber superstars (white beans!), all into a delicious and creamy dish. It's a fantastic way to add some greens and legumes to your diet without any tummy trouble.

Ingredients

- 1 cup cooked white beans (such as cannellini or navy beans), rinsed and drained
- 2 cups fresh spinach leaves
- 1/2 cup low-sodium vegetable broth or water, more if needed for blending
- Salt and pepper to taste
- Optional: A clove of garlic, minced, for added flavor
- Optional: A squeeze of lemon juice for brightness

<u>**Preparation Instructions**</u>

- If using fresh spinach, steam or sauté it until wilted and soft. Allow it to cool.

- In a blender or food processor, combine the cooked white beans, softened spinach, and vegetable broth or water. Start with a smaller amount of liquid and add more as needed to achieve a smooth consistency.

- Add the minced garlic if using, and blend until the mixture is completely smooth. If the puree is too thick, gradually add more broth or water until you reach your desired consistency.

- Season with salt and pepper to taste. Add a squeeze of lemon juice if desired, and blend again briefly to mix.

- Serve the puree warm, or allow it to cool to room temperature if preferred.

<u>**Nutritional Value**</u>

This puree not only offers a good source of plant-based protein from the white beans but also provides iron, calcium, and vitamins A and C from the spinach. It's a balanced dish that supports overall health and recovery.

Nutritional Information

- Calories: Approximately 150-200 per serving
- Protein: 8-10g
- Carbohydrates: 20-25g
- Fat: 1-2g
- Sugar: 2-3g

Expert Tips

- Ensure the beans are thoroughly rinsed and drained if using canned beans to reduce sodium content.
- Adjust the consistency according to your current dietary stage and tolerance, adding more liquid if necessary for a smoother puree.

Cooking Time

20 minutes

The Creamy Spinach and White Bean Puree is a nutritious, flavorful option for those in Phase 3 of the bariatric diet, combining essential proteins, vitamins, and minerals in a dish that's easy on the stomach and delightful to the palate.

Carrot and Ginger Puree

This Carrot and Ginger Puree is a taste bud trip in a bowl. We've blended sweet carrots with a kick of ginger to create a delicious and nutritious puree. Not only is it packed with vitamins and antioxidants, but the ginger can also help with digestion – double win! It's gentle on your tummy but full of good stuff to keep you on track in Phase 3.

Ingredients

- 2 cups carrots, peeled and chopped
- 1-inch piece of fresh ginger, peeled and grated
- 1/2 cup water or low-sodium vegetable broth (for blending)
- Salt to taste
- Optional: A pinch of cinnamon or nutmeg for added warmth and flavor

Preparation Instructions

- Steam the chopped carrots until they are very tender, about 15-20 minutes.
- In a blender or food processor, combine the steamed carrots, grated ginger, and a bit of water or vegetable broth. Start with a small amount of liquid and add more as needed to achieve a smooth, creamy consistency.
- Blend until the mixture is completely smooth. If the puree is too thick, gradually add more liquid until you reach your desired consistency.
- Season with salt to taste, and add a pinch of cinnamon or nutmeg if using, blending again to incorporate.
- Serve the puree warm, or let it cool to room temperature if preferred.

Nutritional Value

Carrots are a great source of beta-carotene, fiber, vitamin K1, potassium, and antioxidants. Ginger adds digestive benefits, helping to soothe the stomach and reduce inflammation. Together, they create a puree that's not only tasty but also supportive of overall health and recovery.

<u>**Nutritional Information**</u>

- Calories: Approximately 70-100 per serving
- Protein: 1-2g
- Carbohydrates: 16-20g
- Fat: 0.2-0.5g
- Sugar: 6-9g

<u>**Expert Tips**</u>

- Make sure the carrots are steamed until they're very soft to ensure a smooth puree, which is easier to digest during this phase of your diet.
- Adjust the amount of ginger according to your taste preferences and tolerance, as it can be quite potent.

<u>**Cooking Time**</u>

25-30 minutes

The Carrot and Ginger Puree is a flavorful, nourishing addition to the Phase 3 bariatric diet, offering a simple way to incorporate more vegetables and spices into your meal plan. Its bright color and soothing properties make it a welcome dish for anyone looking to enjoy a variety of tastes and textures while adhering to dietary guidelines.

Roasted Beet and Apple Puree 

This Roasted Beet and Apple Puree is a flavor explosion in a bowl. We've blended earthy, roasted beets with tart and tangy apples to create a delicious and nutritious puree. It's not just pretty to look at (think vibrant purple!), it's also packed with vitamins and goodness to keep your body thriving. Think of it as a taste bud adventure that fuels you from the inside out – perfect for keeping things interesting in Phase 3!

<u>Ingredients</u>

- 2 medium beets, peeled and cubed
- 2 medium apples, peeled, cored, and chopped (choose a variety with a balance of sweet and tart, like Fuji or Gala)
- 1 tablespoon olive oil (for roasting the beets)
- Water or apple juice, as needed for blending
- Optional: A pinch of cinnamon or ginger for added flavor

<u>**Preparation Instructions**</u>

- Preheat your oven to 400°F (200°C). Toss the cubed beets with olive oil and spread them out on a baking sheet. Roast in the oven for about 30-40 minutes, or until they are tender and easily pierced with a fork.

- Allow the roasted beets to cool slightly. At the same time, steam the chopped apples until they are very soft, about 15-20 minutes.

- In a blender or food processor, combine the roasted beets and steamed apples. Begin blending, adding a small amount of water or apple juice to achieve the desired consistency. The puree should be smooth and free of lumps.

- If using, add a pinch of cinnamon or ginger to the mixture and blend again until the spices are well incorporated.

- Taste and adjust the seasoning, adding more spices if desired. The puree can be served warm or chilled, according to preference.

Nutritional Value

Beets are a great source of fiber, folate (vitamin B9), manganese, potassium, iron, and vitamin C. Apples add additional fiber and vitamin C to the mix, making this puree not only delicious but also very healthful.

Nutritional Information

- Calories: Approximately 100-150 per serving
- Protein: 1-2g
- Carbohydrates: 25-30g
- Fat: 2-3g (from the olive oil)
- Sugar: 18-22g (natural sugars from beets and apples)

Expert Tips

- Roasting beets enhances their natural sweetness, providing a depth of flavor that complements the freshness of the apples.
- Ensure the beets and apples are very soft before blending to achieve a smooth, digestible puree suitable for Phase 3 of the bariatric diet.

- This puree can be stored in an airtight container in the refrigerator for up to 3 days, making it a convenient option for meal prep.

Cooking Time

About 55-60 minutes

The Roasted Beet and Apple Puree is a colorful, nutritious option for those in Phase 3 of the bariatric diet, offering a tasty way to increase your intake of vegetables and fruits while maintaining a smooth texture that's gentle on the digestive system.

Pumpkin and Turkey Puree

This Pumpkin and Turkey Puree is like a fall feast in a bowl. We've blended delicious, protein-packed turkey with creamy pumpkin – a perfect combo for healing and keeping you happy. It's packed with vitamins and fiber from the pumpkin, and lean protein from the turkey to keep your body strong. Think of it as a warm hug on a plate, with a taste of autumn to brighten your day!

Ingredients

- 1 cup cooked turkey breast, finely chopped or shredded
- 1 cup pure pumpkin puree (ensure it's 100% pumpkin, not pie filling)
- 1/2 cup low-sodium chicken broth or water, as needed for blending
- Salt and pepper to taste
- Optional: A pinch of ground cinnamon or nutmeg for added warmth and flavor

<u>**Preparation Instructions**</u>

- If not already cooked, boil or roast the turkey breast until fully cooked, then allow it to cool. Finely chop or shred the meat to ensure smooth blending.

- In a blender or food processor, combine the cooked turkey, pumpkin puree, and a small amount of chicken broth or water. Start with less liquid and add more as needed to achieve a creamy, smooth consistency.

- Season the mixture with salt and pepper. If using, add a pinch of cinnamon or nutmeg to enhance the flavors, blending again to distribute the spices evenly.

- Blend the mixture until completely smooth, adding more broth or water as necessary to reach the desired puree texture.

- Taste and adjust the seasoning if needed. The puree can be served warm, making it a comforting dish for recovery.

<u>**Nutritional Value**</u>

This puree provides a good balance of lean protein from the turkey and carbohydrates from the pumpkin. Pumpkin is also a great source of vitamin A, potassium, and fiber, making this dish not only tasty but also very nutritious.

Nutritional Information

- Calories: Approximately 150-200 per serving
- Protein: 20-25g
- Carbohydrates: 10-15g
- Fat: 1-3g
- Sugar: 2-4g

Expert Tips

Ensure the turkey is cooked thoroughly to make it easier to puree and digest.

Cooking Time

10 minutes

The Pumpkin and Turkey Puree is a nutrient-rich, flavorful option for those in Phase 3 of the bariatric diet, offering a delicious way to meet protein requirements while enjoying the natural sweetness of pumpkin. Its ease of preparation and comforting taste make it an ideal choice for a meal or snack during this phase of recovery.

Salmon and Sweet Potato Puree

This Salmon and Sweet Potato Puree is a flavor and nutrient powerhouse. We've blended delicious salmon, packed with omega-3 goodness, with creamy sweet potatoes for a touch of natural sweetness and vitamins. It's the perfect mix of protein and carbs to keep you feeling full and fueled throughout this phase. Think of it as a taste bud party that nourishes your body from the inside out – delicious and healthy, just what you need in Phase 3!

Ingredients

- 1 cup cooked salmon, skin and bones removed
- 1 cup cooked sweet potato, peeled
- 1/2 cup low-sodium chicken or vegetable broth, as needed for blending
- Salt and pepper to taste
- Optional: A pinch of dill or thyme for added flavor

<u>**Preparation Instructions**</u>

- Ensure the salmon is cooked thoroughly and cooled. Flake the salmon with a fork to remove any skin and bones.

- In a blender or food processor, combine the flaked salmon, cooked sweet potato, and a small amount of broth. Start with less liquid and add more as needed to achieve a smooth, creamy consistency.

- Season the mixture with salt and pepper. If using, add a pinch of dill or thyme to complement the flavors of the salmon and sweet potato.

- Blend until completely smooth, adding more broth as necessary to reach the desired texture. The puree should be free of lumps and easy to eat with a spoon.

- Taste and adjust the seasoning if needed. This puree can be served warm or at room temperature, according to your preference.

<u>**Nutritional Value**</u>

Salmon is an excellent source of high-quality protein and omega-3 fatty acids, which are beneficial for heart health and inflammation reduction. Sweet potatoes contribute fiber, vitamins A and C, and potassium, making this dish a nutritional powerhouse.

Nutritional Information

- Calories: Approximately 200-250 per serving
- Protein: 15-20g
- Carbohydrates: 20-25g
- Fat: 5-10g
- Sugar: 5-7g

Expert Tips

Be sure to remove all skin and bones from the salmon to ensure a smooth puree.

Cooking Time

10 minutes

The Salmon and Sweet Potato Puree is a delicious, nutritious option for individuals in Phase 3 of the bariatric diet. It combines essential nutrients with a creamy texture and rich flavor, making it a satisfying meal choice during the recovery process.

Ricotta and Berry Puree

This Ricotta and Berry Puree is a taste bud adventure in a bowl. We've blended creamy ricotta cheese with a burst of juicy berries for a delicious and refreshing snack or dessert. It's packed with protein from the ricotta and antioxidants from the berries, making it a perfect choice to keep you fueled and on track during recovery. Think of it as a cool and creamy reward that's good for you too – yum!

<u>**Ingredients**</u>

- 1/2 cup low-fat ricotta cheese
- 1/2 cup mixed berries (such as strawberries, blueberries, and raspberries), fresh or frozen and thawed
- A splash of milk or almond milk, if needed for blending
- Optional: A drizzle of honey or a sprinkle of stevia for added sweetness
- Optional: A pinch of vanilla extract for enhanced flavor

<u>**Preparation Instructions**</u>

- If using fresh berries, wash and prepare them by removing any stems or leaves. If using frozen berries, ensure they are fully thawed.

- In a blender or food processor, combine the ricotta cheese, berries, and vanilla extract (if using). Blend on high until the mixture becomes smooth. If the puree is too thick, add a small splash of milk or almond milk to reach the desired consistency.

- Taste the puree and adjust the sweetness if necessary, adding a drizzle of honey or a sprinkle of stevia to your preference. Blend again briefly to incorporate any added sweeteners.

- Serve the puree chilled for a refreshing treat, or at room temperature if preferred.

<u>**Nutritional Value**</u>

This puree offers a good source of protein from the ricotta cheese, essential for muscle repair and overall health during recovery. Berries provide dietary fiber, vitamins, and antioxidants, contributing to a balanced diet.

Nutritional Information

- Calories: Approximately 150-200 per serving
- Protein: 10-14g
- Carbohydrates: 15-20g
- Fat: 4-8g
- Sugar: Natural sugars from the berries

Expert Tips

- Choosing low-fat ricotta cheese helps keep the puree light while still providing a creamy texture.
- Adjust the type and amount of berries according to your personal taste and tolerance levels. Mixing different berries can create a nice blend of flavors and nutrients.

Cooking Time

5 minutes

The Ricotta and Berry Puree is an excellent choice for those in Phase 3 of the bariatric diet, blending rich, smooth ricotta with sweet, nutritious berries for a deliciously simple puree. It's an enjoyable way to include more protein and antioxidants in your diet while satisfying your sweet tooth in a healthy, balanced manner.

Lentil Soup Puree

Our Lentil Soup Puree takes classic lentil soup and blends it into a smooth, creamy dream. It's super nourishing, warming on a chilly day, and oh-so-satisfying. Plus, it's easy on your tummy, making it perfect for this stage of your journey. Think of it as a cozy hug in a bowl, packed with all the good stuff your body needs to thrive!

Ingredients

- 1 cup cooked lentils (preferably soft cooked)
- 2 cups low-sodium vegetable broth or water
- 1/2 cup diced carrots, cooked until very soft
- 1/2 cup diced celery, cooked until very soft
- 1 small onion, sautéed until translucent
- Salt and pepper to taste
- Optional: Garlic, thyme, or bay leaves for added flavor (remove bay leaves before blending)

<u>**Preparation Instructions**</u>

- If starting with uncooked lentils, rinse them thoroughly and boil until they are very soft and almost falling apart. Drain and set aside.

- In a large pot, combine the cooked lentils, soft-cooked carrots, celery, and sautéed onion. Add the vegetable broth or water. If you're using garlic or herbs for additional flavor, add them to the pot as well.

- Bring the mixture to a gentle simmer and let it cook for about 10-15 minutes, allowing the flavors to meld together. Remove from heat and let it cool slightly.

- Carefully remove any bay leaves or large herb stems. Transfer the mixture to a blender or use an immersion blender directly in the pot.

- Blend the soup until it achieves a smooth, creamy consistency. If the puree is too thick, add a bit more broth or water until you reach your desired texture.

- Season with salt and pepper to taste, and blend again briefly to incorporate.

- Serve the puree warm, or allow it to cool to room temperature if preferred.

Nutritional Value

This lentil soup puree is rich in plant-based protein and dietary fiber, which are essential for maintaining muscle health and supporting digestive health, respectively. The vegetables add vitamins and minerals, making this a well-rounded, nutritious meal.

Nutritional Information

- Calories: Approximately 150-200 per serving
- Protein: 10-15g
- Carbohydrates: 25-30g
- Fat: 1-2g
- Sugar: 3-5g

Expert Tips

- Ensure the lentils and vegetables are cooked until very soft to achieve a smooth puree that's easy to digest.

- Adjust the seasoning and herbs according to your taste preferences, keeping in mind that your sense of taste may be more sensitive during recovery.

- This puree can be stored in the refrigerator for up to 3 days, making it a convenient make-ahead meal option.

Cooking Time

30-45 minutes

The Lentil Soup Puree is an excellent choice for anyone in Phase 3 of the bariatric diet, offering a tasty, nutritious way to incorporate legumes and vegetables into your diet in a form that's gentle on the digestive system. Its comforting flavor and nutritional benefits make it a satisfying meal or side dish.

Chapter 5

Phase 4: The Soft Foods Diet

Welcome to Phase 4, the grand finale of your bariatric diet phases! This is where you take everything you've learned about mindful eating and apply it to a wider variety of foods. It's like the final act of a play, where all the characters come together, and the story reaches its peak.

Phase 4 typically begins around week 8 post-surgery and is all about stabilization and maintenance. You've navigated through the clear liquids, embraced the protein shakes, and mashed your way through purees. Now, it's time to enjoy foods of regular consistency, but with a newfound respect for balance and portion control.

Here's what Phase 4 is all about:

- **Balanced Meals:** You'll be eating three well-portioned, nutrient-rich meals a day. We're talking lean meats, low-fat dairy, whole grains, fruits, and veggies. It's like a colorful palette of options, each providing the nutrients your body needs to thrive.

- **Protein First:** Protein remains the star, so start your meals with it. Whether it's chicken, fish, or tofu, make sure you're getting enough to support your body's healing and energy needs.

- **Mindful Eating:** Continue to eat slowly and listen to your body's fullness cues. It's about savoring every bite and recognizing when you've had just enough.

- **Hydration:** Keep up with your fluids, but remember to drink between meals, not during. This helps prevent stretching your stomach and ensures you're getting the most out of your meals.

- **Snack Smart:** If you need a little something between meals, reach for a protein shake or a small, healthy snack. It's about making choices that align with your goals.

- **Vitamins and Supplements:** Since your meals are smaller, you'll likely continue with supplements to meet your daily nutritional needs.

As you settle into Phase 4, it's all about making this sustainable. You're creating a lifestyle that includes a variety of foods, but in a way that maintains your weight loss and health improvements. It's not just a phase; it's the beginning of your new life.

So, here's to the foods that nourish you, the habits that sustain you, and the life you're building with every mindful choice. Welcome to your new normal!

Flaky Poached Fish

Welcome to Phase 4! Time to introduce some yummy, soft foods back into your routine. Flaky Poached Fish is your new best friend – it's packed with protein that your body loves, but super gentle on your tummy. Plus, poaching keeps the fish moist and delicious, making it the perfect way to ease back into eating soft foods. Think of it as a protein party for your body, with a light and fluffy texture that won't overwhelm you!

Ingredients

- 1 fillet of mild white fish (such as cod, tilapia, or sole), about 6 ounces
- 2 cups low-sodium vegetable or fish broth
- Optional: Lemon slices and fresh dill or parsley for flavoring
- Salt and pepper to taste

<u>**Preparation Instructions**</u>

- In a deep skillet or saucepan, bring the broth to a gentle simmer over medium heat. If using, add lemon slices and fresh dill or parsley to the broth to infuse it with additional flavors.
- Season the fish fillet lightly with salt and pepper. Carefully place the fish in the simmering broth. The broth should cover or nearly cover the fish.
- Cover the skillet or saucepan with a lid and let the fish poach at a gentle simmer for about 6-10 minutes, depending on the thickness of the fillet. The fish is done when it flakes easily with a fork.
- Using a slotted spatula, carefully remove the fish from the broth and plate it. The fish should be moist and flaky.
- Garnish with additional fresh herbs if desired. Serve immediately, ensuring the fish is soft and easily broken apart with a fork.

<u>**Nutritional Value**</u>

These wraps are a powerhouse of lean protein, courtesy of the turkey. The lettuce and veggies chip in with vitamins and minerals, supporting your well-being with every bite.

Nutritional Information

- Calories: Approximately 100-150 per serving
- Protein: 20-25g
- Carbohydrates: 0-1g
- Fat: 1-3g
- Sugar: 0g

Expert Tips

- Ensure the broth is at a gentle simmer before adding the fish to prevent it from falling apart.
- Poaching is a moist cooking method that helps keep the fish tender and prevents it from drying out, ideal for those in Phase 4 of the bariatric diet.

Cooking Time

About 15-20 minutes, including preparation and cooking time.

Flaky Poached Fish is a simple, nutritious dish well-suited for the soft foods phase of the bariatric diet. Its gentle cooking method and delicate texture make it an excellent choice for reintroducing more solid proteins into your diet while ensuring ease of digestion and enjoyment.

Scrambled Eggs with Spinach

Scrambled Eggs with Spinach is a breakfast (or anytime!) dream. Fluffy eggs give you a protein boost, while the spinach sneaks in some iron, fiber, and vitamins – all the good stuff! It's super easy to make and gentle on your tummy, making it perfect for this stage of your journey. Think of it as a delicious way to fuel your body and keep your recovery rolling!

Ingredients

- 2 large eggs
- 1 cup fresh spinach leaves, washed and roughly chopped
- 1 tablespoon low-fat milk or water (for fluffier eggs)
- Salt and pepper to taste
- Optional: A pinch of grated low-fat cheese for added flavor
- Optional: A dash of turmeric or paprika for color and health benefits. A sprinkle of fresh herbs, like cilantro or mint, to garnish (optional but recommended)

Preparation Instructions

- In a bowl, whisk the eggs with the low-fat milk or water until well combined. Season with salt and pepper.
- Heat a non-stick skillet over medium-low heat. Add the chopped spinach and sauté for 1-2 minutes until it begins to wilt.
- Pour the egg mixture over the spinach in the skillet. Let it sit for a moment before gently stirring with a spatula to form soft curds.
- Continue cooking, stirring occasionally, until the eggs are fully cooked but still moist and fluffy. Avoid overcooking to maintain a soft texture.
- If using, sprinkle a pinch of grated low-fat cheese on top of the eggs just before they're finished cooking, allowing it to melt.
- Serve the scrambled eggs warm, optionally garnished with a dash of turmeric or paprika for extra flavor and color

Nutritional Value

This dish is rich in protein, essential for healing and muscle maintenance, and provides a good dose of leafy greens, offering iron, magnesium, and vitamins A, C, and K. It's a balanced, healthful meal that supports your dietary goals in Phase 4.

<u>**Nutritional Information**</u>

- Calories: Approximately 150-200 per serving
- Protein: 12-16g
- Carbohydrates: 2-4g
- Fat: 10-14g (mostly healthy fats from the eggs)
- Sugar: 1-2g

<u>**Expert Tips**</u>

- Cooking the eggs on medium-low heat helps prevent them from becoming rubbery, ensuring they stay soft and fluffy.
- Adding a small amount of milk or water to the eggs can help create a lighter texture.

<u>**Cooking Time**</u>

10 minutes

Scrambled Eggs with Spinach is a nutritious, simple dish suited for Phase 4 of the bariatric diet. It combines the wholesome goodness of eggs and spinach in a meal that's both satisfying and easy to digest, perfect for those advancing towards more solid foods in their diet.

Ricotta Bake

Our Ricotta Bake is like a warm hug on a plate. We use creamy, low-fat ricotta cheese and bake it with yummy herbs until it's just set. It's soft, comforting, and packed with protein, making it a delicious and gentle way to keep your body happy during this phase.

Ingredients

- 1 cup low-fat ricotta cheese
- 1 large egg, lightly beaten
- 2 tablespoons grated Parmesan cheese
- Salt and pepper to taste
- Optional: Fresh herbs (such as basil, parsley, or chives), finely chopped, for added flavor
- Optional: A pinch of garlic powder for a flavor boost

<u>**Preparation Instructions**</u>

- Preheat your oven to 350°F (175°C). Lightly grease a small baking dish with cooking spray or a bit of olive oil.
- In a mixing bowl, combine the low-fat ricotta cheese, beaten egg, and grated Parmesan cheese. Mix well until the ingredients are fully incorporated.
- Season the mixture with salt and pepper. If using, fold in the chopped fresh herbs and garlic powder to add depth to the flavor.
- Pour the ricotta mixture into the prepared baking dish, smoothing the top with a spatula.
- Bake in the preheated oven for about 20-25 minutes, or until the mixture is set and the top is slightly golden.
- Allow the Ricotta Bake to cool for a few minutes before serving. It can be enjoyed warm or at room temperature.

<u>**Nutritional Value**</u>

This Ricotta Bake is an excellent source of calcium and high-quality protein from the ricotta and Parmesan cheeses, supporting bone health and muscle repair. The addition of egg not only helps set the bake but also adds to its protein content.

Nutritional Information

- Calories: Approximately 200-250 per serving
- Protein: 14-18g
- Carbohydrates: 4-6g
- Fat: 12-16g
- Sugar: 2-4g

Expert Tips

- Adding fresh herbs not only enhances the flavor but also increases the nutritional value with additional vitamins and antioxidants.
- This dish can be customized with various seasonings and herbs to match your taste preferences or to complement other dishes.

Cooking Time

30 minutes

The Ricotta Bake is a versatile, nutrient-rich dish perfect for those in Phase 4 of the bariatric diet. Its creamy texture and comforting taste make it a delightful choice for breakfast, a snack, or even a light meal, offering a pleasant way to meet your protein needs while enjoying a flavorful, soft food option.

Mashed Sweet Potatoes with Cinnamon

Sweet potatoes are loaded with vitamins, fiber, and even antioxidants, while the cinnamon adds a cozy touch (and might even help with your sugar levels!). This dish is naturally sweet, creamy, and super easy on your tummy – perfect for this stage of your journey.

Ingredients

- 2 medium sweet potatoes, peeled and cubed
- 1/4 cup low-fat milk or almond milk
- 1 tablespoon unsalted butter or coconut oil (for a dairy-free option)
- 1/2 teaspoon ground cinnamon
- Salt to taste
- Optional: A drizzle of honey or a sprinkle of nutmeg for additional sweetness and flavor

<u>**Preparation Instructions**</u>

- Place the cubed sweet potatoes in a large pot and cover with water. Bring to a boil over high heat, then reduce to a simmer. Cook until the sweet potatoes are very tender, about 15-20 minutes.
- Drain the sweet potatoes and return them to the pot or a large mixing bowl. Add the low-fat milk, butter or coconut oil, and ground cinnamon.
- Mash the sweet potatoes with a potato masher or blend with an immersion blender until smooth and creamy. Adjust the consistency with more milk if needed.
- Season with salt to taste. If desired, add a drizzle of honey or a sprinkle of nutmeg for extra sweetness and spice.
- Serve warm, garnished with a little extra cinnamon on top for presentation.

<u>**Nutritional Value**</u>

Sweet potatoes are an excellent source of beta-carotene, which the body converts to vitamin A, essential for eye health and immunity. The added cinnamon not only enhances flavor but also offers health benefits, including anti-inflammatory properties and blood sugar regulation.

Nutritional Information

- Calories: Approximately 150-200 per serving
- Protein: 2-3g
- Carbohydrates: 35-40g
- Fat: 2-4g (varies depending on the choice of butter or oil)
- Sugar: Natural sugars from the sweet potatoes, with optional added honey

Expert Tips

- Cooking the sweet potatoes until they're very tender ensures a smooth, creamy texture that's easier to mash and digest.
- Using low-fat milk or a dairy-free alternative like almond milk keeps the dish lighter while still providing creaminess.

Cooking Time

About 25-30 minutes

Mashed Sweet Potatoes with Cinnamon is a delightful, nutritious option for those in Phase 4 of the bariatric diet, offering a sweet and comforting dish that's rich in vitamins and easy on the stomach.

Avocado Chicken Salad

Avocado Chicken Salad is like a flavor fiesta in a bowl. We've combined creamy avocado with tender chicken for a dish that's soft, easy to eat, and packed with goodness. The avocado adds some heart-healthy fats, while the chicken gives you a protein boost – it's a win-win for your taste buds and your body!

Ingredients

- 1 cup cooked chicken breast, finely shredded
- 1 ripe avocado, pitted and mashed
- 1/4 cup Greek yogurt (for added creaminess and protein)
- Salt and pepper to taste
- Optional: A squeeze of lemon juice to prevent the avocado from browning and add a tangy flavor
- Optional: Fresh herbs such as cilantro or parsley, finely chopped, for additional flavor

<u>**Preparation Instructions**</u>

- Ensure the chicken breast is cooked thoroughly and cooled. Using a fork, finely shred the chicken into small pieces suitable for easy digestion.

- In a mixing bowl, combine the mashed avocado and Greek yogurt, mixing until smooth and well-blended.

- Add the shredded chicken to the avocado mixture. Stir until the chicken is fully coated and the ingredients are evenly distributed.

- Season the salad with salt and pepper to taste. If using, add a squeeze of lemon juice and the chopped fresh herbs, mixing well to incorporate.

- Chill the salad in the refrigerator for about 30 minutes before serving, or serve immediately if preferred.

<u>**Nutritional Value**</u>

This salad is a fantastic source of lean protein, essential for muscle repair and maintenance, and monounsaturated fats, beneficial for heart health. The addition of Greek yogurt not only enhances the creaminess of the dish but also adds a probiotic boost.

Nutritional Information

- Calories: Approximately 250-300 per serving
- Protein: 20-25g
- Carbohydrates: 8-12g
- Fat: 15-20g
- Sugar: 2-4g

Expert Tips

- Opt for low-fat Greek yogurt to keep the dish light while still creamy.

- Lemon juice not only adds flavor but also helps in keeping the avocado from turning brown, preserving the salad's fresh, vibrant color.

Cooking Time

30 minutes

Avocado Chicken Salad is an excellent meal choice for those in Phase 4 of the bariatric diet, blending the nutritional benefits of avocado and chicken in a soft, flavorful dish. It's ideal for a light lunch or a satisfying snack, offering both taste and texture that are well-suited for this stage of dietary progression.

Soft Baked Salmon with Herbs

Soft Baked Salmon with Herbs is like a fancy restaurant dish you can make at home. Salmon is super good for you, packed with protein and those amazing omega-3 fatty acids. We bake it nice and soft with delicious herbs, making it perfect for this phase of your journey. It's tasty, nutritious, and gentle on your tummy.

Ingredients

- 2 salmon fillets (about 6 ounces each)
- 1 tablespoon olive oil
- Salt and pepper to taste
- A mix of fresh herbs (such as dill, parsley, or thyme), finely chopped
- Optional: Lemon slices for garnish and added flavor

Preparation Instructions

- Preheat your oven to 350°F (175°C). Line a baking sheet with parchment paper or lightly grease it with a bit of olive oil.

- Place the salmon fillets on the prepared baking sheet. Brush each fillet lightly with olive oil and season with salt and pepper.

- Sprinkle the chopped herbs evenly over the salmon fillets. If using, place a few lemon slices on top for extra moisture and flavor during baking.

- Bake in the preheated oven for about 12-15 minutes, or until the salmon is cooked through and flakes easily with a fork. The exact time may vary depending on the thickness of the fillets.

- Once done, carefully remove the salmon from the oven and let it rest for a few minutes before serving. This allows the juices to redistribute, ensuring the salmon remains moist and flavorful.

Nutritional Value

Salmon is an excellent source of omega-3 fatty acids, which are essential for heart health, brain function, and inflammation reduction. It's also rich in high-quality protein, vitamins D and B, and selenium.

Nutritional Information

- Calories: Approximately 200-250 per serving
- Protein: 22-25g
- Carbohydrates: 0g
- Fat: 12-15g
- Sugar: 0g

Expert Tips

- Keeping the salmon moist is key to a soft texture. The olive oil and lemon slices help achieve this by locking in moisture during baking.
- Be careful not to overcook the salmon to maintain its soft, flaky texture, which is easier to digest at this stage of your diet.

Cooking Time

15-20 minutes

Soft Baked Salmon with Herbs is a beautifully simple, nutritious dish suitable for Phase 4 of the bariatric diet. It combines the health benefits of salmon with the fresh flavors of herbs, creating a meal that's both satisfying and supportive of your dietary progression and overall health.

Quinoa and Vegetable Stew

Quinoa and Vegetable Stew is soft and filling, and it's a complete protein powerhouse! We've added a bunch of colorful veggies for vitamins, minerals, and fiber. This stew is perfectly balanced, nutritious, and gentle on your tummy – the perfect way to keep things interesting and delicious in Phase 4!

Ingredients

- 1/2 cup quinoa, rinsed
- 2 cups low-sodium vegetable broth
- 1 cup diced carrots, cooked until very soft
- 1 cup diced zucchini, cooked until very soft
- 1/2 cup diced tomatoes (canned or fresh, with juices)
- 1 teaspoon olive oil
- Salt and pepper to taste
- Optional: Fresh herbs (such as thyme or parsley) for flavoring

Preparation Instructions

- In a medium pot, heat the olive oil over medium heat. Add the rinsed quinoa and toast for 1-2 minutes, stirring frequently.
- Add the low-sodium vegetable broth to the pot and bring to a boil. Reduce the heat to low, cover, and simmer for about 15 minutes, or until the quinoa is cooked and most of the liquid is absorbed.
- Stir in the cooked carrots, zucchini, and diced tomatoes (with juices) into the pot with the quinoa. If using, add the fresh herbs at this point.
- Continue to simmer the stew for another 5-10 minutes, allowing the flavors to meld together and the vegetables to become tender.
- Season the stew with salt and pepper to taste. Adjust the consistency by adding more broth if needed.
- Serve the stew warm, ensuring it's thoroughly cooked and the vegetables are soft enough to meet the dietary requirements of Phase 4.

Nutritional Value

This stew is rich in plant-based protein from quinoa, which also provides essential amino acids. The variety of vegetables ensures a broad spectrum of vitamins and minerals, supporting overall health and recovery.

Nutritional Information

- Calories: Approximately 200-250 per serving
- Protein: 8-10g
- Carbohydrates: 35-40g
- Fat: 3-5g
- Sugar: 5-7g

Expert Tips

- Ensure the vegetables are diced small and cooked until very soft to make them easier to digest.

- Quinoa is a versatile grain that absorbs flavors well, so feel free to customize this stew with your favorite vegetables or herbs.

Cooking Time

30 minutes

Quinoa and Vegetable Stew is a hearty, flavorful dish ideal for those in Phase 4 of the bariatric diet. It's designed to provide a comforting meal that's easy on the digestive system while still offering the nutritional benefits needed for recovery and health maintenance.

Cottage Cheese Pancakes

Cottage Cheese Pancakes are like fluffy clouds packed with protein. We've blended creamy cottage cheese into delicious pancakes that are soft, easy to chew, and oh-so-satisfying. They're a perfect way to enjoy a yummy meal or snack during this phase, all while keeping your tummy happy and your protein goals on track.

Ingredients

- 1/2 cup low-fat cottage cheese
- 2 large eggs
- 1/4 cup all-purpose flour or almond flour for a lower-carb option
- 1 tablespoon sugar or a sugar substitute for a lower-calorie option
- 1/2 teaspoon baking powder
- 1/2 teaspoon vanilla extract
- A pinch of salt
- Optional: A dash of cinnamon or nutmeg for added flavor

<u>**Preparation Instructions**</u>

- In a blender or food processor, combine the cottage cheese, eggs, flour, sugar (or sugar substitute), baking powder, vanilla extract, and a pinch of salt. Blend until the mixture is smooth.
- Heat a non-stick skillet or griddle over medium heat. Lightly grease it with a small amount of butter or oil.
- Pour small amounts of the batter onto the skillet to form pancakes. Cook for 2-3 minutes on one side or until bubbles form on the surface and the edges look set.
- Carefully flip the pancakes and cook for an additional 1-2 minutes on the other side until golden brown and cooked through.
- Serve the pancakes warm, optionally topped with a dollop of Greek yogurt or a drizzle of sugar-free syrup for added moisture and flavor.

<u>**Nutritional Value**</u>

Cottage Cheese Pancakes offer a good balance of proteins and carbohydrates, with the cottage cheese providing a high-quality protein source that's essential for muscle repair and recovery. The addition of eggs increases the protein content and nutritional value, making these pancakes both satisfying and healthful.

<u>**Nutritional Information**</u>

- Calories: Approximately 200-250 per serving (depending on the type of flour and sugar used)
- Protein: 15-20g
- Carbohydrates: 20-25g
- Fat: 5-10g
- Sugar: 2-5g

<u>**Expert Tips**</u>

For those sensitive to dairy or looking to reduce carbohydrate intake, almond flour and a sugar substitute can be used as alternatives to all-purpose flour and sugar.

<u>**Cooking Time**</u>

15 minutes

Cottage Cheese Pancakes are a versatile, delicious option for anyone in Phase 4 of the bariatric diet. Their soft texture, combined with the nutritional benefits of cottage cheese and eggs, makes them an ideal choice for reintroducing more solid foods into the diet while keeping meals interesting and flavorful.

Turkey and Sweet Potato Shepherd's Pie

Ditch the bland and say hello to the Turkey and Sweet Potato Shepherd's Twist! This ain't your grandma's recipe (although she'd probably approve). We've taken the classic shepherd's pie and given it a healthy makeover. It's lean, protein-packed, and guaranteed to satisfy your taste buds without weighing down your tummy. Perfect for when you're ready to level up your meals in Phase 4, but still crave that feel-good comfort food magic.

Ingredients

- 1 lb ground turkey (lean)
- 2 cups mashed sweet potatoes (prepared from cooked and mashed sweet potatoes, with a bit of low-fat milk and seasoning)
- 1 cup diced carrots, cooked until very soft
- 1 cup frozen peas, thawed
- 1 onion, finely chopped
- 2 cloves garlic, minced

- 1/2 cup low-sodium chicken or vegetable broth

- 1 tablespoon olive oil

- Salt and pepper to taste

- Optional: A pinch of thyme or rosemary for added flavor

Preparation Instructions

- Preheat your oven to 375°F (190°C).

- In a large skillet, heat the olive oil over medium heat. Add the chopped onion and minced garlic, sautéing until the onion is translucent.

- Add the ground turkey to the skillet, breaking it apart with a spoon. Cook until the turkey is no longer pink and is fully cooked through.

- Stir in the cooked carrots and thawed peas, along with the low-sodium chicken or vegetable broth. Bring to a simmer and let cook for a few minutes until the mixture is slightly thickened. Season with salt, pepper, and optional herbs.

- Transfer the turkey and vegetable mixture into a baking dish, spreading it out evenly.

- Spoon the mashed sweet potatoes over the turkey mixture, spreading it out to cover completely.

- Bake in the preheated oven for 20-25 minutes, or until the sweet potato topping starts to brown slightly.

- Let the shepherd's pie cool for a few minutes before serving. It should be warm and the layers well set for easy serving.

Nutritional Value

This dish is rich in protein from the ground turkey, essential for muscle repair, and high in vitamins A and C from the sweet potatoes, supporting immune health and vision. The vegetables add fiber and additional nutrients, making it a balanced meal option.

Nutritional Information

- Calories: Approximately 300-350 per serving
- Protein: 20-25g
- Carbohydrates: 35-40g
- Fat: 10-15g
- Sugar: 5-10g

<u>**Expert Tips**</u>

- Ensure the carrots are cooked until very soft to maintain a texture suitable for Phase 4 of the bariatric diet.

- The mashed sweet potatoes should be creamy but not too liquidy to prevent the pie from becoming soggy.

- This dish can be made in advance and reheated, making it a convenient option for meal prep during the week.

<u>**Cooking Time**</u>

45-60 minutes

Turkey and Sweet Potato Shepherd's Pie is a comforting, nutritious dish ideal for Phase 4 of the bariatric diet. It offers a tasty, satisfying meal that adheres to dietary guidelines while providing a mix of lean protein, vegetables, and a healthy carb source, making it a great option for reintroducing more solid foods into your diet.

Pumpkin Apple Puree

We've got a taste bud trip waiting for you in a bowl - the Pumpkin Apple Power Up! Forget bland purees, this is a flavor explosion that celebrates the best of autumn. We've blended creamy pumpkin with bursts of sweet apple, creating a soft and delicious treat that's packed with vitamins and fiber. It's like a warm hug for your tummy, helping you conquer Phase 4 with a smile (and a satisfied taste for pumpkin spice magic).

Ingredients

- 1 cup canned pumpkin puree (ensure it's 100% pumpkin, not pie filling)
- 2 medium apples, peeled, cored, and chopped
- 1/2 teaspoon ground cinnamon
- 1/4 teaspoon ground nutmeg
- Optional: A splash of water or apple juice to adjust consistency
- Optional: A drizzle of honey or maple syrup for added sweetness, if desired

Preparation Instructions

- In a medium saucepan, add the chopped apples with a small amount of water. Cover and cook over medium heat until the apples are very soft and beginning to break down, about 10-15 minutes.

- Add the cooked apples to a blender or food processor, along with the canned pumpkin puree. Blend until smooth. If the mixture is too thick, add a splash of water or apple juice to reach your desired consistency.

- Season the puree with cinnamon and nutmeg, blending again to incorporate the spices evenly.

- Taste the puree and, if desired, add a small drizzle of honey or maple syrup for extra sweetness. Blend briefly to mix.

- Serve the puree warm, or allow it to cool to room temperature before serving, based on your preference.

Nutritional Value

This puree is a great source of dietary fiber and vitamins A and C, thanks to the pumpkin and apples. The spices not only add flavor but also offer additional health benefits, including anti-inflammatory properties.

Nutritional Information

- Calories: Approximately 100-150 per serving
- Protein: 1-2g
- Carbohydrates: 25-30g
- Fat: 0.5-1g
- Sugar: Natural sugars from the apples, with optional added honey or maple syrup

Expert Tips

- Cooking the apples until they are very soft ensures a smooth puree, ideal for the soft foods phase of the diet.
- Using canned pumpkin puree saves time and ensures a consistent texture, but make sure it's unsweetened and unflavored.

Cooking Time

30 minutes

Pumpkin Apple Puree is a flavorful, nutritious option suitable for Phase 4 of the bariatric diet. Its combination of sweet and spice offers a comforting taste experience, making it a versatile dish that can be enjoyed as a snack, dessert, or even a side dish.

Bonus Chapter

10 Easy Herbal Tinctures & Smoothies to Speed up Your Recovery

Step into the cozy kitchen of recovery, where each blend and brew is a toast to your vibrant health. In this special bonus chapter, we're going to mix up a little magic with ten easy recipes for herbal tinctures and smoothies that'll soothe, nourish, and invigorate you as you heal from your VSG.

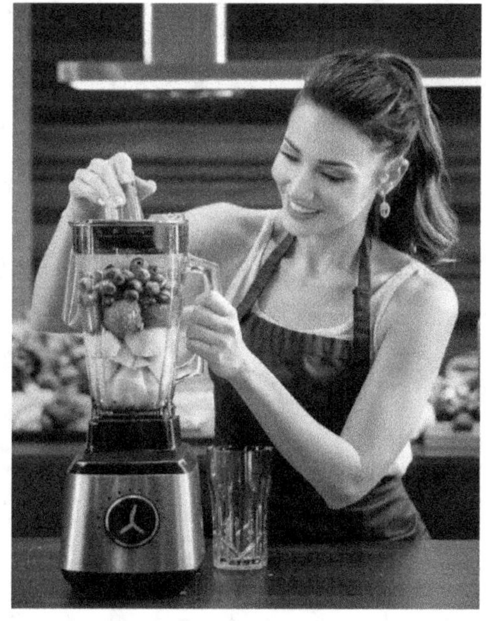

Imagine each recipe as a handwritten note from a friend, filled with care and crafted to bring a smile to your face. These aren't just drinks; they're liquid hugs, infused with the healing power of herbs and the pure joy of fruits and veggies. They're your daily dose of deliciousness that'll help speed up your recovery, one sip at a time.

So, pull up a chair, grab your favorite cup, and let's blend up some comfort. Whether it's the gentle embrace of chamomile or the cheerful zing of ginger, these tinctures and smoothies are your companions on the journey to feeling like your best self again. Here's to finding joy in the simple things and savoring every moment of your journey back to health.

Ginger Tincture

This isn't your grandma's ginger tea (although grandma might be impressed). We're talking about a ginger extract so powerful, it'll turn your tummy into a chill zone. Feeling nauseous after surgery? Ginger Warrior to the rescue! Just a few drops in some water or tea, and you'll be feeling soothed and satisfied. It's like a superhero for your tummy, helping you conquer post-surgery recovery like a champ!

Ingredients

- 1 cup fresh ginger root, finely chopped or grated
- 2 cups high-proof alcohol (such as vodka or grain alcohol, at least 80 proof to ensure preservation and extraction)
- Optional: A drizzle of honey or maple syrup for added sweetness, if desired

<u>**Preparation Instructions**</u>

- Thoroughly wash the ginger root and pat it dry. Peel the ginger, then finely chop or grate it to increase the surface area for better extraction.

- Place the chopped or grated ginger in a clean, dry jar. Pour the alcohol over the ginger until it's completely submerged.

- Seal the jar tightly and label it with the date. Store the jar in a cool, dark place.

- Shake the jar daily to help the extraction process. Allow the mixture to steep for 4 to 6 weeks. The longer it sits, the stronger your tincture will be.

- After the steeping period, strain the tincture through a fine-mesh sieve or cheesecloth into another clean, dry jar or bottle. Press or squeeze the ginger pulp to extract as much liquid as possible.

- Discard the ginger pulp and transfer the strained tincture to a dark glass dropper bottle for easy use and storage.

<u>**Nutritional Value**</u>

Ginger contains gingerol, a substance with powerful anti-inflammatory and antioxidant effects. This tincture concentrates those properties, making them readily available in a form that's easy to dose and consume as part of a post-operative recovery plan.

<u>**Expert Tips**</u>

- If you prefer a non-alcoholic version, glycerin can be used as an alternative to alcohol, though the preservation properties and extraction efficacy may vary.

- Start with small doses of the tincture to gauge your tolerance, especially if you're sensitive to ginger's potent effects. A typical dose might start from a few drops to a teaspoon, diluted in water or tea.

Ginger Tincture is a simple yet effective way to incorporate the digestive and anti-inflammatory benefits of ginger into your post-VSG recovery diet. It's a versatile remedy that can be adjusted to fit individual needs and preferences, providing a natural option for managing digestive health and inflammation.

Turmeric Tincture

Tired of boring pills? Meet your new best friend, the Turmeric Torch Tincture! This isn't your average kitchen spice. We're talking about a concentrated dose of turmeric goodness, packed with curcumin, a superhero molecule that fights inflammation and keeps your joints happy. But wait, there's more! This tiny tincture is also an antioxidant powerhouse, helping your body fight free radicals and recover like a champ. Just a few drops in water or your favorite tea, and you'll be feeling the vibrant glow of turmeric magic. Ditch the drugstore routine and unlock the ancient power of turmeric with the Turmeric Torch Tincture!

Ingredients

- 1 cup fresh turmeric root, finely chopped or grated (alternatively, you can use dried turmeric root)
- 2 cups high-proof alcohol (such as vodka or grain alcohol, at least 80 proof to ensure proper extraction and preservation)

<u>**Preparation Instructions**</u>

- Clean the turmeric root thoroughly and pat it dry. Peel the root and finely chop or grate it. If using dried turmeric, ensure it's broken down into small pieces to maximize the surface area for extraction.
- Place the turmeric in a clean, dry jar. Pour the alcohol over the turmeric until it is fully submerged.
- Seal the jar tightly with a lid and label it with the date. Store the jar in a cool, dark place, away from direct sunlight.
- Shake the jar daily to mix the contents and promote extraction. Allow the mixture to steep for 4 to 6 weeks. The longer it steeps, the more potent the tincture will become.
- After the steeping period, strain the liquid through a fine-mesh sieve or cheesecloth into another clean, dry jar or bottle, squeezing out as much liquid as possible.
- Discard the turmeric solids and transfer the tincture to a dark glass dropper bottle for storage and easy dosing.

Nutritional Value

Turmeric's main active component, curcumin, offers significant anti-inflammatory properties and acts as a strong antioxidant. This tincture provides a concentrated form of curcumin, making its beneficial effects more readily available for absorption.

Expert Tips

- Sterilize all jars and utensils before use to ensure the tincture remains uncontaminated.
- Begin with a low dosage, such as a few drops, to assess tolerance, as turmeric can be potent. It can be taken directly under the tongue or diluted in a small
- Including a bit of black pepper in the tincture can enhance the absorption of curcumin by the body, thanks to the compound piperine found in black pepper.

Turmeric Tincture is a valuable addition to a post-VSG recovery plan, offering an easy way to benefit from the anti-inflammatory and antioxidant properties of turmeric. This homemade tincture can be a versatile part of your wellness routine, adaptable to your individual health needs and preferences.

Chamomile Tincture

We've captured the calming magic of chamomile flowers in a tiny bottle, making it your secret weapon for a relaxed recovery. Feeling stressed after surgery? Chamomile Chill to the rescue! This little potion is a natural remedy for anxiety and digestive woes, helping you unwind and drift off to sleep with ease. So ditch the sleep aids and embrace the power of nature with Chamomile Chill Tincture

Ingredients

- 1 cup dried chamomile flowers
- 2 cups high-proof alcohol (such as vodka or grain alcohol, at least 80 proof, to ensure effective extraction and preservation)

Preparation Instructions

- Place the dried chamomile flowers in a clean, dry jar. If you're using fresh chamomile flowers, ensure they are completely dry to prevent mold growth in the tincture.

- Pour the alcohol over the chamomile flowers until they are fully submerged. Stir gently to ensure all the flowers are soaked in alcohol.

- Seal the jar tightly with a lid. Label the jar with the current date for reference.

- Store the jar in a cool, dark place, such as a cupboard or pantry. Shake the jar gently once a day to agitate the flowers and aid in the extraction process.

- Allow the mixture to steep for 4 to 6 weeks. The longer it steeps, the stronger and more potent the tincture will become.

- After steeping, strain the tincture through a fine-mesh sieve or cheesecloth into a clean, dry bottle or jar. Press or squeeze the chamomile flowers to extract as much liquid as possible.

- Transfer the strained tincture to a dark glass dropper bottle for storage and easy use. Discard the used chamomile flowers.

Nutritional Value

Chamomile is widely recognized for its mild sedative effects, which can help improve sleep quality and relaxation. It also possesses anti-inflammatory and antispasmodic properties, making it beneficial for soothing digestive troubles.

Expert Tips

- Make sure all equipment is sterilized before starting to avoid contamination.
- Start with a small dose, such as a few drops in water or tea, to assess your tolerance and response to the tincture, especially if you are new to herbal remedies.
- Store the tincture in a cool, dark place to preserve its potency. Properly stored, a tincture can last for several years.

Chamomile Tincture is a gentle, natural remedy ideal for enhancing relaxation and supporting digestive health during the recovery phase post-VSG. Its preparation is straightforward, offering a convenient way to enjoy the benefits of chamomile in a concentrated, easy-to-use form.

Peppermint Tincture

Say hello to your new BFF, the Peppermint Powerhouse Tincture! This isn't your average breath mint. We're talking about a concentrated dose of peppermint magic, specifically designed to tame a troubled tummy. Feeling nauseous? Peppermint Powerhouse to the rescue! This little bottle packs a punch against indigestion and discomfort, leaving you feeling refreshed and clear-headed. Just a few drops in some water or tea, and you'll be back on your feet and feeling minty fresh in no time. Skip the bland remedies and unleash the power of peppermint with the Peppermint Powerhouse Tincture – your tummy will thank you for it!

Ingredients

- 1 cup fresh peppermint leaves (or 1/2 cup dried peppermint leaves)
- 2 cups high-proof alcohol (such as vodka or grain alcohol, at least 80 proof, to ensure effective extraction and preservation)

<u>**Preparation Instructions**</u>

- If using fresh peppermint leaves, rinse them thoroughly and pat dry. Roughly chop the leaves to increase the surface area for extraction.

- Place the peppermint leaves in a clean, dry jar. If using dried leaves, ensure they're crumbled or roughly chopped.

- Pour the alcohol over the leaves until they are fully submerged. Use a spoon to stir gently, making sure all the leaves are soaked in alcohol.

- Seal the jar with a tight-fitting lid. Label the jar with the date to keep track of the steeping duration.

- Store the jar in a cool, dark place, shaking it gently every day to facilitate the extraction process.

- Allow the mixture to steep for 3 to 4 weeks. The steeping time can be adjusted based on the desired potency.

- After steeping, strain the tincture through a fine-mesh sieve or cheesecloth into a clean, dry container. Compress the peppermint leaves to extract as much liquid as possible.

- Transfer the strained tincture to a dark glass dropper bottle for convenient storage and dosing. Dispose of the used peppermint leaves properly.

Nutritional Value

Peppermint is known for its menthol content, which can help relax the muscles of the digestive tract, reducing symptoms of indigestion and irritable bowel syndrome. It's also appreciated for its invigorating scent that can help boost energy and mental alertness.

Expert Tips

- Sterilize your equipment before use to prevent contamination.
- Fresh peppermint leaves will yield a more vibrant tincture, but dried leaves are also effective and can be stored and used year-round.
- A small dose is usually sufficient to experience the benefits of the tincture. It can be taken directly under the tongue or diluted in a small amount of water or tea.

- Store your tincture in a cool, dark place to maintain its potency. When stored properly, it can last for several years.

Peppermint Tincture is a versatile and powerful herbal remedy suitable for easing digestive discomfort and supporting overall well-being during the recovery phase after VSG surgery. Its refreshing flavor and therapeutic properties make it a valuable addition to your post-surgery care regimen.

Milk Thistle Tincture

Meet Milk Thistle Max, your liver's new best friend! This tiny bottle is packed with silymarin, a powerful shield that protects your liver cells and helps them regenerate like tiny champions. Milk Thistle Max is also an antioxidant powerhouse, helping your body fight off free radicals and bounce back even stronger. Think of it as a magic potion for your liver, helping it work its best and get you feeling on top of the world again. Just a few drops a day, and your liver will be thanking you for the TLC!

Ingredients

- 1 cup milk thistle seeds, crushed or ground (to maximize extraction of silymarin)
- 2 cups high-proof alcohol (such as vodka or grain alcohol, at least 80 proof, to ensure proper extraction and preservation)

<u>**Preparation Instructions**</u>

- Begin by crushing or grinding the milk thistle seeds to open them up and improve the extraction process. A mortar and pestle or a coffee grinder can be used for this purpose.
- Place the ground milk thistle seeds in a clean, dry jar.
- Pour the alcohol over the seeds, ensuring they are completely submerged. Stir gently to mix.
- Seal the jar tightly with a lid and label it with the date to keep track of the steeping time.
- Store the jar in a cool, dark place. Shake the jar daily to agitate the seeds and facilitate the extraction of silymarin.
- Allow the mixture to steep for 4 to 6 weeks. The longer it steeps, the stronger the tincture will be.
- After the steeping period, strain the tincture through a fine-mesh sieve or cheesecloth into another clean, dry container, squeezing or pressing to extract as much liquid as possible.
- Transfer the strained tincture to a dark glass dropper bottle for storage and easy use. Discard the milk thistle solids.

<u>**Nutritional Value**</u>

Milk thistle is celebrated for its liver-protective qualities, particularly due to silymarin, which has antioxidant, antiviral, and anti-inflammatory properties. This tincture offers a concentrated form of these benefits, supporting liver detoxification and health.

<u>**Expert Tips**</u>

- Crushing or grinding the milk thistle seeds is crucial for a potent tincture as it exposes more surface area to the alcohol for extraction.
- If you're sensitive to alcohol, the tincture can be added to hot water to evaporate some of the alcohol before consumption.

Milk Thistle Tincture is a thoughtful addition to a post-VSG recovery plan, aimed at supporting liver function and overall health. Its preparation is straightforward, offering a natural, powerful tool for enhancing liver detoxification and protection during the recovery journey.

Protein-Packed Green Smoothie

Ditch the medicine cabinet and unleash the power of nature with this potent ginger extract. We're talking about a ginger warrior so fierce, it'll calm your tummy and soothe nausea faster than you can say "ouch!". Just a few drops in water or tea, and you'll be feeling like your old, nausea-free self in no time. This natural remedy is your secret weapon for a smooth recovery – conquer post-surgery like a champ, with the power of Mother Earth on your side!

Ingredients

- 1 cup fresh spinach leaves
- 1/2 cup low-fat Greek yogurt
- 1 scoop vanilla or unflavored protein powder
- 1/2 a medium cucumber, chopped
- 1/2 a green apple, cored and chopped
- Water or almond milk, as needed for blending
- Ice cubes (optional, for a colder smoothie)

<u>**Preparation Instructions**</u>

- Add the spinach leaves, Greek yogurt, protein powder, chopped cucumber, and green apple to a blender. If you're using a protein powder, choose one that complements or enhances the natural flavors of the smoothie ingredients.

- Begin blending on a low setting, gradually adding water or almond milk until you achieve your desired consistency. The amount of liquid needed can vary depending on how thick or thin you prefer your smoothie.

- Once the ingredients start to combine, increase the blender speed to high and blend until the smoothie is completely smooth and all components are fully incorporated. For a colder, more refreshing drink, add ice cubes to the blend.

- Taste the smoothie, and adjust the sweetness if necessary. Depending on the protein powder used, you may want to add a small amount of honey or a sugar substitute.

- Serve the smoothie immediately, garnishing with a small sprig of fresh mint or a few slices of cucumber for an extra touch of freshness.

Nutritional Value

This smoothie is rich in protein from the Greek yogurt and protein powder, essential for muscle repair and growth. Spinach and cucumber provide a good source of vitamins A, C, K, magnesium, and iron, while the green apple adds dietary fiber and additional vitamin C.

Nutritional Information

- Calories: Approximately 100-150 per serving
- Protein: 1-2g
- Carbohydrates: 25-30g
- Fat: 0.5-1g
- Sugar: Natural sugars from the apples, with optional added honey or maple syrup

Expert Tips

- Using cold ingredients or adding ice cubes makes the smoothie more refreshing, especially after a workout or on a hot day.

- If you're sensitive to dairy or prefer a vegan option, plant-based protein powder and non-dairy yogurt alternatives can be used.

- Customizing your smoothie with different leafy greens like kale or adding other non-starchy vegetables can vary the nutrient profile and flavor.

The Protein-Packed Green Smoothie is a versatile, nutritious option for anyone in the later stages of the bariatric diet or maintaining a healthy lifestyle post-surgery. It's a simple way to boost your protein intake while enjoying the health benefits of fresh vegetables and fruits.

Berry Antioxidant Smoothie

Buckle up, because the Berry Blaster Smoothie is here to fuel your transformation! This vibrant drink packs a punch of antioxidants from juicy berries, plus protein and omega-3 goodness from chia seeds. Blended with creamy almond milk, it's a taste bud party in a glass and a total win for your health. Blast off your mornings with this delicious smoothie, or grab it for an afternoon pick-me-up. It's a nutritious and revitalizing reward for your amazing journey!

Ingredients

- 1 cup mixed berries (such as strawberries, blueberries, raspberries), fresh or frozen
- 1 tablespoon chia seeds
- 1 cup unsweetened almond milk (or any other plant-based milk of your choice)
- 1 scoop of your preferred protein powder (optional, for an extra protein boost)
- Ice cubes (optional, for added chill and texture)

<u>**Preparation Instructions**</u>

- If using fresh berries, rinse them well. If opting for frozen berries, there's no need to thaw them as they help create a chilled, thick smoothie.

- Place the berries, chia seeds, almond milk, and protein powder (if using) in a blender.

- Blend on high until the mixture is smooth and creamy. Depending on your blender's power and whether you're using frozen berries, this might take a minute or two.

- If the smoothie is too thick for your liking, add a little more almond milk to reach your desired consistency. If you prefer your smoothie colder or thicker, add a few ice cubes and blend again.

- Once the smoothie has reached your preferred consistency and smoothness, taste it. If you find it needs a bit more sweetness, consider adding a natural sweetener like stevia or a splash of honey, then blend briefly to incorporate.

- Serve the smoothie immediately, garnished with a few whole berries on top for a beautiful and appetizing presentation.

<u>**Nutritional Value**</u>

This smoothie is packed with antioxidants from the berries, which can help neutralize free radicals and reduce inflammation. Chia seeds add fiber, protein, and omega-3 fatty acids, making the smoothie even more satisfying and beneficial for heart health. Adding protein powder can further support muscle repair and growth.

<u>**Nutritional Information**</u>

- Calories: Approximately 150-250, depending on the addition of protein powder and the type of milk used
- Protein: 10-20g (with protein powder)
- Carbohydrates: 20-30g
- Fat: 4-8g
- Sugar: Natural sugars from the berries

<u>**Expert Tips**</u>

- Using frozen berries can give the smoothie a refreshing chill and a thicker consistency, reminiscent of a sorbet or ice cream.

- Chia seeds not only thicken the smoothie but also provide a time-released form of hydration as they absorb liquid and expand.
- Personalize your smoothie by mixing and matching different types of berries to find your favorite combination or to take advantage of what's in season.

The Berry Antioxidant Smoothie is a delightful, health-boosting beverage ideal for anyone in Phase 4 of the bariatric diet or anyone looking to enhance their diet with antioxidant-rich, flavorful foods. Its combination of taste and nutrition makes it a perfect choice for supporting your health and recovery journey.

Golden Turmeric Smoothie

The Golden Glow Getter Smoothie is your secret weapon for inner and outer radiance. This sunshine-colored drink is packed with the magic of turmeric, known for its anti-inflammatory and antioxidant powers. We've blended it with creamy banana for a touch of sweetness and rich coconut milk for a taste bud vacation. It's not just delicious, it's a functional food powerhouse that perfectly complements your Phase 4 journey, or anyone looking for a daily dose of wellness. Drink your way to a healthier, happier you – sip by sip!

Ingredients

- 1 large ripe banana
- 1 cup coconut milk (unsweetened, for a creamy texture and tropical flavor)
- 1 teaspoon ground turmeric (increase to taste, considering turmeric's potent flavor)
- A pinch of black pepper (to enhance curcumin absorption)

- 1 scoop of vanilla or unflavored protein powder (optional, for added protein)

- A dash of cinnamon or nutmeg (for extra warmth and complexity)

- Ice cubes (optional, for a thicker and colder smoothie)

Preparation Instructions

- Peel the banana and break it into chunks. Place the banana pieces into a blender.

- Add the coconut milk to the blender, ensuring it's unsweetened to keep the smoothie as healthful as possible.

- Sprinkle in the ground turmeric and a pinch of black pepper. The pepper is critical as it contains piperine, which significantly boosts the bioavailability of curcumin from turmeric.

- If using protein powder, add it to the blender along with your choice of cinnamon or nutmeg for additional flavor.

- Add a few ice cubes if you prefer your smoothie cold and thick.

- Blend on high until the mixture is smooth and creamy. If the smoothie is too thick, you can add a little more coconut milk or water to reach your desired consistency.

- Taste the smoothie and adjust the sweetness or spices to your liking. If you prefer a sweeter smoothie, you might add a touch of honey or maple syrup, then blend again to mix.

Nutritional Value

Turmeric is renowned for its anti-inflammatory and antioxidant properties, which can support recovery and overall health. Coconut milk provides healthy fats, while banana offers natural sweetness, potassium, and dietary fiber. Adding protein powder makes this smoothie a more complete meal, especially beneficial for muscle repair and satiety.

Nutritional Information

- Calories: Approximately 200-300, depending on the use of protein powder and the type of coconut milk
- Protein: 10-20g (with protein powder)

- Carbohydrates: 20-30g
- Fat: 5-15g
- Sugar: 10-15g (natural sugars from the banana)

Expert Tips

- Fresh turmeric root can be used in place of ground turmeric for a more potent flavor and health benefits. Just a small piece, about an inch, peeled and chopped, will suffice.

- The inclusion of black pepper is crucial for enhancing the absorption of curcumin, so don't skip it!

- Adjust the amount of turmeric according to your tolerance, as it has a strong flavor that not everyone is accustomed to.

The Golden Turmeric Smoothie is an excellent way to start your day or recharge your afternoon with a dose of powerful antioxidants and anti-inflammatory compounds. This smoothie is not just a treat for your taste buds but a boost for your health, perfectly aligning with the nutritional needs of those in Phase 4 of the bariatric diet.

Ginger-Peach Soothing Smoothie

This refreshing drink combines the tummy-taming power of ginger with the sweet, juicy goodness of peaches. It's like a spa day in a glass, gentle enough for Phase 4 but packed with flavor and anti-inflammatory benefits. Plus, it's a delicious way to support your digestion and overall well-being.

Ingredients

- 1 cup fresh or frozen peaches (if using fresh, ensure they are ripe and sweet)
- 1 small piece (about 1 inch) of fresh ginger, peeled and grated
- 1/2 cup low-fat vanilla yogurt (to add creaminess and probiotics)
- 1 teaspoon honey (optional, adjust based on the sweetness of the peaches)
- Water or almond milk, as needed for blending
- Ice cubes (optional, for a cooler, thicker smoothie)

<u>**Preparation Instructions**</u>

- If using frozen peaches, there's no need to thaw them as they'll help create a chilled, thick smoothie. For fresh peaches, wash, pit, and slice them.
- Place the peaches, grated ginger, and vanilla yogurt into a blender. The ginger adds a spicy, warming note that complements the sweetness of the peaches, while the yogurt brings a smooth, creamy texture to the smoothie.
- Add a splash of water or almond milk to help the ingredients blend smoothly. Start with a small amount and add more as needed to achieve your desired consistency.
- Blend on high until the mixture becomes smooth. If the smoothie is too thick, add a little more liquid and blend again.
- Taste the smoothie and, if desired, add honey for extra sweetness. Blend again briefly to incorporate any added sweeteners.
- If you prefer a colder beverage, add a few ice cubes and blend until smooth.

- Serve the smoothie immediately, garnishing with a thin slice of peach or a sprinkle of ground ginger on top for a decorative touch.

Nutritional Value

Ginger is known for its ability to aid digestion and reduce nausea, making it an excellent choice for soothing the stomach. Peaches provide dietary fiber, vitamins (such as Vitamin C and A), and antioxidants. The addition of low-fat yogurt not only enhances the texture but also introduces probiotics, beneficial for gut health.

Nutritional Information

- Calories: Approximately 150-200 per serving
- Protein: 5-10g (depending on the type of yogurt used)
- Carbohydrates: 20-30g
- Fat: 0.5-2g
- Sugar: Natural sugars from the peaches and honey

<u>**Expert Tips**</u>

- Adjust the amount of ginger based on your preference for spice and its digestive benefits. Fresh ginger tends to be more potent than dried.

- For those lactose intolerant or preferring a dairy-free option, a plant-based vanilla yogurt can be used in place of traditional dairy yogurt.

- This smoothie can be customized with additional fruits or a scoop of protein powder to increase its nutritional content.

The Ginger-Peach Soothing Smoothie is a delightful blend of flavors and health benefits, making it a perfect addition to your dietary routine in Phase 4 of the bariatric diet. Its combination of natural sweetness with a hint of spice offers a refreshing way to support digestion and overall wellness.

Healing Herbal Smoothie

Recovery got you feeling like you need a little green magic? The Green Glow-Up Smoothie is your answer! This revitalizing drink is packed with nature's healers, all blended into a delicious concoction. We're talking soothing aloe vera, hydrating cucumber and parsley, and a tangy twist of green apple and lemon juice. It's a detoxifying dream team in a glass, perfect for Phase 4 or anyone looking for a daily dose of wellness.

Ingredients

- 1/2 cup aloe vera juice (ensure it's pure and suitable for internal use)
- 1 small cucumber, peeled and chopped
- 1/2 cup fresh parsley leaves
- 1 green apple, cored and chopped
- Juice of 1/2 lemon
- Water or coconut water, as needed for blending
- Ice cubes (optional, for added chill)

<u>**Preparation Instructions**</u>

- Start by preparing the ingredients: wash the cucumber, parsley, and green apple. Peel the cucumber if it's not organic to reduce pesticide exposure. Chop the cucumber and apple into pieces small enough to blend smoothly.

- In a blender, combine the aloe vera juice, chopped cucumber, parsley leaves, chopped green apple, and lemon juice. The aloe vera juice is known for its healing properties, while cucumber and parsley offer hydration and detoxification benefits. The green apple and lemon add a natural sweetness and tanginess, as well as additional vitamins.

- Add a splash of water or coconut water to help the ingredients blend more easily. Start with a small amount, adjusting as needed to achieve your preferred smoothie consistency.

- Blend on high until the mixture is completely smooth. If you like your smoothie colder or thicker, add a few ice cubes and blend again.

- Taste the smoothie and adjust the flavor as needed. If it's too tart, you might add a small amount of honey or agave syrup to sweeten.

- Serve the smoothie immediately, enjoying the fresh, invigorating flavors and the health benefits it provides.

Nutritional Value

This smoothie is packed with vitamins, minerals, and antioxidants from its fresh ingredients. Aloe vera juice can help support gastrointestinal health, while cucumber and parsley are great for hydration and detoxification. Green apple and lemon juice add a boost of vitamin C and other antioxidants, supporting immune function and skin health.

Nutritional Information

- Calories: Approximately 100-150 per serving
- Protein: 1-2g
- Carbohydrates: 20-25g
- Fat: Less than 1g
- Sugar: Natural sugars from the apple and optional sweetener

<u>**Expert Tips**</u>

- Ensure the aloe vera juice you use is labeled for internal use, as some aloe products are intended for topical use only.

- Adjusting the amount of lemon juice can help balance the smoothie's sweetness and tartness to your liking.

- This smoothie can serve as a refreshing morning beverage or a soothing drink to enjoy any time of day when you need a hydrating and healing boost.

The Healing Herbal Smoothie is a light, refreshing option ideal for those in the later stages of recovery from bariatric surgery, providing a blend of ingredients known for their supportive and restorative properties. It's a wonderful way to incorporate more hydrating and detoxifying elements into your diet while enjoying a delicious, health-promoting drink.

Conclusion

As we reach the final pages of our shared story, I want to sit with you for a moment, from one heart to another. This book was a journey we embarked on together, a path paved with hope, nourishment, and the promise of a new beginning.

Through the chapters, you've discovered the gentle guidance of the bariatric diet, the courage that comes with embracing the VSG, and the careful steps of the four diet stages that have been your companions in this transformation. Each recipe, each piece of advice, was a token of my wish for your well-being.

And then, there was the bonus chapter, a little gift wrapped in the warmth of herbal tinctures and the freshness of smoothies, each one a whisper of comfort to speed you on your way to recovery.

Now, I wonder, have these pages been a friend to you? Have you found within them the answers you were seeking, the solace for your questions? It's my deepest hope that this book has been a lantern in the night, guiding you through the shadows to a place of health and happiness.

As you close this book and continue your journey, remember that you walk with a legion of souls who know your struggle, who cheer for your victories, and who share in the silent understanding of what it means to seek a better life.

May your recovery be swift, may your spirit be light, and may you always know that in the quiet moments when doubt whispers, you are never, ever alone.

With all the warmth in my heart,

Catherine D. Crisp.

Thank you for purchasing and reading this book. I sincerely hope that you have found the solution to your problem. If you have enjoyed reading this book, please leave a kind review so others can find the book and also get the help they need.

Also below, are a books you will enjoy reading.

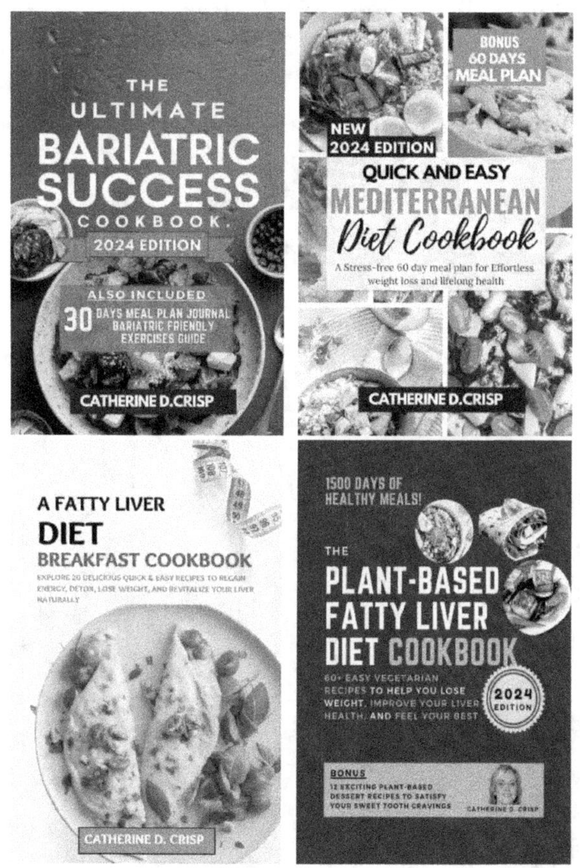

All titles are available on Amazon.

Before you go, I would like to ask a personal favor from you. Writing this book took a lot of time and effort as I wanted to make this the best possible guide for you as you explore the different recipes through your Bariatric diet and VSG recovery.

This meant countless hours of research and compilation to ensure that within these pages, you find the resources you need and the answers to your questions.

So dear friend, I will like to kindly ask you to leave a review of the book so that others with similar questions or needs can find this book and get the help they need from within its pages.

I really appreciate looking forward to your kind reviews.

Love and light

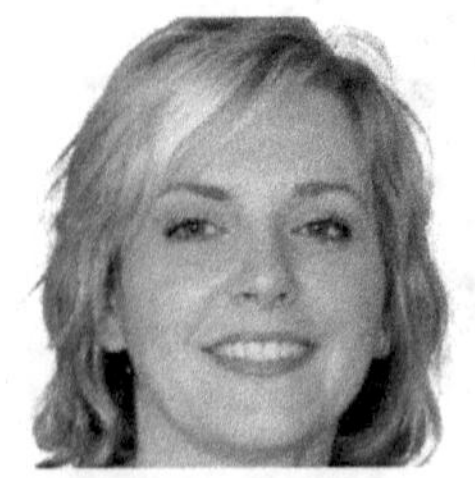

Catherine D Crisp.